MW01030680

OnlineMedEd

www.onlinemeded.org

For information about permission to use or reproduce selections from this book, email help@onlinemeded.org with the subject, "Additional QuickTables Usage."

Authored by Dustyn Williams and Jamie Fitch
Produced by Staci Weber
Covers designed by Aaron Root

ISBN 978-0-9969501-1-4

Published by OnlineMedEd, www.onlinemeded.org

Printed in the United States of America

2nd Edition

This is a review book; if you haven't learned the material already, it may be confusing and generate a lot of questions. If you use this book after reading the notes, watching the videos, and doing the Qbank, you'll better understand its purpose.

It's meant to be used for repetition and reinforcement—highlighting buzz phrases and key elements of each disease. Read this over several times in a block or during shelf/step studying to lock in the facts you'll need.

You can read it BEFORE you engage the lectures as a way to prime yourself, but it won't make any sense; it'll look like gibberish that doesn't connect. It's better to read AFTER you engage the lessons (our intent). You can't remember everything about everything—this will help you spot key elements in vignettes and wade through extraneous information. The more you read it—the more repetitions—the easier the test will be.

Again, this isn't meant to be a reference book—you SHOULD NOT learn from it. But it takes very little to engage it, which means you can pull it out whenever you have downtime. It doesn't require a studying groove or a large time commitment to get into it.

We've tried to leave a lot of WHITE SPACE. That's so you can put in notes as you study. Remember the purpose and make them brief. Each time you read through the QuickTables you'll also be reading notes to yourself, so add what you need to help with your repetition/interests.

This is the second edition. We've combed through it pretty hard and had thousands of students before you vet it. But, it still may not be perfect—we make typos, recommendations change, and new findings come out. If you spot an error, let us know so we can tell everyone else and make the third edition even better.

— Dustyn and Jamie

Table of Contents

Coronary Artery Disease

MYOCARDIAL INFARCTION	
Path:	Occlusion of a coronary vessel
Pt:	Chest pain that is worse with exertion, better with rest, relieved with nitrates in a hypertensive, diabetic, dyslipidemic smoker, who is old
Dx:	ST segment changes = STEMI Biomarker Elevation = NSTEMI Stress Test = CAD Coronary Angiogram = best test
Tx:	Morphine, Oxygen, Nitrates, Aspirin (MONA) β-blocker, ACE-inhibitor, Statin, Heparin (BASH) Coronary Angiography with Stent (single vessel disease) CABG (multi-vessel disease) tPA if no transport available (60 minutes)

RISK FACTORS AND GOALS	
Hypertension	< 140 / < 90
Diabetes	A1c < 7.0
Smoking	Cessation
Dyslipidemia	LDL < 100, better < 70 HDL > 40, better > 60
Age	Woman > 55 Man > 45

STORY	PHYSICAL
Left sided / Substernal	Nonpositional
Worse with exertion	Nonpleuritic
Better with rest	Nontender

	STABLE ANGINA	UNSTABLE ANGINA	NSTEMI	STEMI
Pain	Exercise	@ rest	@ rest	@ rest
Relief	Rest + Nitrates	∅	∅	∅
Trops	∅	∅	↑	↑
ST Δs	∅	∅	∅	↑

ACUTE TREATMENT OPTIONS	
ASA	FIRST drug to give
Nitrates	Second
Angioplasty	No clopidogrel needed, only in single-vessel disease
Bare-Metal Stent	Clopidogrel x 1 month, only in single-vessel disease
Drug-Eluting Stent	Clopidogrel x 1 year, only in single-vessel disease
CABG	Left Mainstem equivalent or multi-vessel disease
tPA	No PCI is available within 60 minutes transport time
Door-to-balloon	90 minutes
	Prasugrel = Clopidogrel

CHRONIC TREATMENT OPTIONS	
β-blocker	BP < 140 / < 90, HR < 70
ACE-inhibitor	BP < 140 / < 90
Aspirin	Antiplatelet
Clopidogrel	Antiplatelet
Statins	LDL < 100 (prefer < 70)

STRESS TESTING	
Imaging	
EKG	Test of choice, no baseline abnormality
Echo	EKG abnormalities, no CABG
Nuclear	CABG, Baseline wall defects, LBBB
Testing	
Exercise	Test of choice, no contraindication to exercise with feet
Pharm	Any reason why they can't get on a treadmill, of any kind. Dobutamine and Adenosine essentially identical

COMPLICATIONS OF MI	
RV Failure	Right Sided ECG No Nitrates
Aneurysm	Diagnosed by Echo
Arrhythmia	VTach / VFib—ventricular ectopy from dying cells Brady / Blocks—AV nodal dysfunction

Congestive Heart Failure

SIDED HEART FAILURE	
Left Sided	Pulmonary Edema, Shortness of breath, Crackles, Dyspnea on exertion, Orthopnea, Paroxysmal nocturnal dyspnea, S3
Right Sided	JVD, Peripheral Edema, Abdominal pain

SYSTOLE vs. DIASTOLE	
Systole	Floppy (ischemic / chronic), leaky (valves), or dead (ischemic) Depressed ejection fraction Poor forward flow
Diastole	Stiff ventricle, unable to fill Pericardium (tamponade, constrictive pericarditis) Restrictive or Hypertrophic Cardiomyopathy

NYHA	
I	No symptoms, unlimited exertional capacity
II	Slight Limitation: comfortable with exertion and rest, but without unlimited capacity
III	Moderate Limitation: comfortable at rest only
IV	Severe Limitations, patient is dyspneic at rest

DIAGNOSTIC CHOICES	
CXR	Large heart, generally useless
ECG	Old ischemia, generally useless
BNP	If elevated, likely heart failure, but cannot discern left/right, diastolic/systolic
2D Echo	Test of choice, gives much information including EF and diastolic failure, valve lesions
Nuclear	Gives EF and reversible ischemia
Angiogram, LVgram	Gold Standard, invasive, generally not needed
Angiogram, Coronaries	Determine CAD state: ischemic cardiomyopathy vs. not

TREATMENT	
Everybody	β-blocker, ACE-inhibitor Salt Restrict < 2g NaCl Fluid Restrict < 2L H2O
Ischemic	Add Aspirin, Add Statin
EF < 35%	AICD

TREATMENT BY NYHA STAGE			
I	BB + ACE		
II		Loop Diuretics	
III			BiDil Spirono
IV	↓	↓	↓ Pressors

BiDil = Hydralazine / Isosorbide DiNitrate
BB = β-blocker, ACE = ACE-inhibitor
Spirono = Spironolactone / Eplerenone

CONGESTIVE HEART FAILURE	
Path:	Systolic vs. Diastolic Right vs. Left Ischemic vs. Non-Ischemic
Pt:	Dyspnea on exertion, Paroxysmal Nocturnal Dyspnea, Orthopnea. Peripheral Edema, Crackles, JVD
Dx:	1st: BNP Then: 2D Echo = Transthoracic Echo Best: LV Ventriculogram
Tx:	Systolic: NYHA Stage Diastolic: Control BB

CONGESTIVE HEART FAILURE EXACERBATION	
Path:	Ischemia, Arrythmia, Diet Noncompliance, Medication Noncompliance
Pt:	Dypsnea, Worsening orthopnea, anything on the above patient presentation
Dx:	BNP (elevations = exacerbations) ECG and Troponins (etiology) 2D Echo not necessary on each exacerbation
Tx:	Lasix (furosemide) IV Morphine (research debating utility) Nitrates Oxygen Position (upright)

Valve Disease

GRADING VALVES	
Grade	Findings
I	S1, S2 > Murmur (murmur is softer)
II	S1, S2 = Murmur (murmur is equal)
III	S1, S2 < Murmur (murmur is louder)
IV	Palpable thrill
V	1/2 stethoscope off chest, still audible
VI	No stethoscope is needed
	Investigate any diastolic murmur and any systolic murmur ≥ 3/6 (more than II) Use 2D echo to evaluate all murmurs
	TEE better, but often not needed Cath is the best test, can give actual numerical evaluations

MITRAL STENOSIS	
Path:	Rheumatic heart disease, stenosis of valve Decreased forward flow during **diastole** Atrial stretch
Pt:	AFib with CHF symptoms Opening Snap Diastolic Decrescendo Murmur
Dx:	Echo
Tx:	Balloon Valvotomy Valve replacement ~~Commissurotomy~~ (not anymore)

AORTIC STENOSIS	
Path:	Calcification, Sclerosis of outflow from ventricle
Pt:	Old men with atherosclerosis Shortness of breath, Syncope, chest Pain Crescendo-Decrescendo murmur 2nd intercostal space, right sternal border
Dx:	Echo
Tx:	Valve replacement Balloon doesn't work (can be palliative) ~~Know the word TAVR and TAVI~~
F/u:	CABG assessment if replacing valves

MITRAL VALVE PROLAPSE	
Path:	Congenital defect
Pt:	Women, especially pregnant Sounds like Mitral Regurg, opening snap More Blood = Less Murmur
Dx:	Echo
Tx:	Valve replacement

MITRAL REGURGITATION	
Path:	Acute = Infarction, Infection, Ruptured Papillary Muscle, Chordae Tendinae Chronic = Prolapse, Ischemia
Pt:	Acute = Fulminant CHF, Hypoxemia, Hypotension, Chronic = AFib, Exertional Dyspnea, HOLOSYSTOLIC murmur, radiating to the axilla
Dx:	Echo
Tx:	Valve Replacement

AORTIC INSUFFICIENCY (REGURG)	
Path:	Ischemia, Infection, Dissection
Pt:	Usually sick, hypotension, CHF Decrescendo Murmur at Aortic Valve Wide Pulse Pressure Water-Hammer Pulses (Bounding) Quincke's Pulse (Nailbeds) Head bobbing
Dx:	Echo
Tx:	Valve Replacement Intra-Aortic Balloon Pump

HYPERTROPHIC OBSTRUCTIVE CARDIOMYOPATHY	
Path:	Sarcomere Defect
Pt:	Sudden Cardiac Death Dyspnea, Syncope with exertion YOUNG patient
Dx:	Echo
Tx:	Avoid exercise β-blockade Myotomy

Cardiomyopathy

DILATED CARDIOMYOPATHY	
Path:	↓ Contractility Virus, EtOH, Ischemia, Chemo

Pt:	Systolic CHF:
	     Orthopnea, PND, DOE
	     Crackles, Dyspnea, JVD

Dx:	Echo = Dilated

Tx:	CHF: BB, ACE-I, Diuretics
	     Avoid / Stop EtOH
	     Avoid / Stop Chemo
	     Transplant

HOCM	
Path:	Genetics, Sarcomeres

Pt:	Murmur = Aortic Stenosis
	 Young Athletes
	     - Sudden Cardiac Death
	     - Syncope
	     - Dypsnea on Exertion

Dx:	Echo = Asymmetric
Tx:	Avoid Dehydration Avoid Exercise BB = CCB EtOH Ablation, Myectomy AICD for ↑ Risk of death Transplant

CONCENTRIC HYPERTROPHIC CARDIOPMYOPATHY	
Path:	HTN
Pt:	Diastolic CHF
Dx:	Echo = Concentric

Tx:	DIA CHF
	     Avoid Dehydration
	     CCB = BB
	     Control BLOOD PRESSURE
	 Transplant

RESTRICTIVE CARDIOMYOPATHY	
Path:	Amyloid, Sarcoid, Hemachromatosis, Cancer and Fibrosis
Pt:	DIA CHF Amyloid → Neuropathy Sarcoid → Pulmonary Disease Hema → Cirrhosis, Diabetes, CHF
Dx:	Echo = Restrictive Amyloid → Fat Pad Biopsy Sarcoid → Cardiac MRI → Biopsy Hema → Ferritin → Genetics
Tx:	DIA CHF BB = CCB Gentle Diuresis Transplant Underlying Disease

Pericardial Disease

ETIOLOGIES OF PERICARDIAL DISEASE	
Infxn	** Viral **, Bacterial, Fungal, TB
AI	RA, LSA, Dressler's, * Uremia **
Trauma	Penetrating, Blunt Aortic Dissection
Cancer	Breast, Lung, Esophageal, Lymphoma

TREATMENTS	
Pericarditis	Anti-Inflammatories
Effusion	Pericardial Window
Tamponade	Pericardiocentesis
Constrictive	Pericardiectomy
F/u:	Pericardial Window if refractory

PERICARDITIS	
Path:	Viral, Uremia
Pt:	Chest Pain = Pleuritic and Positional

Dx:	1st: ECG shows
	    PR depressions
	    Diffuse ST elevations
	~~Echo~~
	Best: MRI

Tx:	NSAIDS + Colchicine NSAIDS—CKD, ↓ Plt, PUD Colchicine—Diarrhea ~~Steroids~~
F/u:	↑ Recurrence after steorids Hemodialysis for Uremia

PERICARDIAL EFFUSION	
Path:	Pericarditis
Pt:	Pericarditis
Dx:	Echo = Effusion
Tx:	Pericarditis
F/u:	Pericardial Window if refractory

PERICARDIAL TAMPONADE	
Path:	RV cannot fill
Pt:	JVD + Hypotension + ↓ Heart Sounds (Beck's Triad) Clear Lungs Pulsus Paradoxus > 10mmHg
Dx:	Echo
Tx:	Pericardiocentesis ~~Pericardial Window~~ (too slow)
F/u:	IVF in IRL

CONSTRICTIVE PERICARDITIS	
Path:	Pericarditis
Pt:	Diastolic CHF Pericardial Knock
Dx:	Echo
Tx:	Pericardiectomy

Hypertension

	HYPERTENSION MEDICATIONS	
Class	*Side Effect*	*Indications*
CCB	Peripheral Edema	JNC8, Angina
ACE	↑ K, Cough, Angioedema	JNC8
ARB	↑ K, NO cough NO angioedema	ACE-I
Thiazide	↓ K, Urine Sxs	GFR > 60
Loop	↓ K, Urine Sxs	GFR < 60
BB	↓ HR	CAD, CHF
Art - Dilator	Reflex Tachycardia	CHF
Veno - Dilator	Sildenafil = Hypotension	CHF
Spiron - Olactone	↑ K, Gynecomastia	CHF
Clonidine	* Rebound HTN *	Never

	HYPERTENSION
Pt:	120/80 is normal 140/90 is Stage I 160/100 is Stage II

Dx:	Screen EVERYONE
	    2 readings
	    2 weeks
	    2 visits
	Best: Ambulatory Monitoring

Tx:	See above

	STAGES OF HTN (JNC-7)		
Stage	*Sys BP*	*Dia BP*	*Meds*
Normal	120	80	Lifestyle
Pre-HTN			Lifestyle
Stage I	140	90	1 med
Stage II	160	100	2 med
Urgency	180	110	Orals
Emergency	End Organ Damage		IVs

	JNC-8 GUIDELINES
1	> 60 and NO disease = 150/90
2	Everyone Else = 140/90
3	CCB, Thiazide, ACE/ARB are ok
4	Old and Black = no ACE/ARB
5	CKD = ACE/ARB
6	No β-blockers!! (4th med)

If old, black, and no CKD . . . no ACE/ARB.

Cholesterol

CHOLESTEROL	
Path:	Need enough to make cells Too much makes plaques Plaques make atherosclerosis
Pt:	HDL is the "good" cholesterol LDL is the "bad" cholesterol Non-HDL Cholesterol is what matters
Dx:	Lipid Panel
Tx:	Diet and Exercise is always first Adherence
F/u:	Statins . . . Others

STATINS		
Drug	Good Effect	Bad Effect
Statin	↓ LDL, ↓ TG	Myositis ↑ LFT
Fibrates	↓ Tchol, ↑ HDL	Myositis ↑ LFT
Ezetimibe	↓ LDL	Diarrhea *
Bile-Acid Resins	↓ LDL	Diarrhea
Niacins	↑ HDL, ↓ LDL	Flushing ASA

WHO GETS A STATIN?	
1)	Vascular Disease (CVA, PVD, CAD)
2)	LDL ≥ 190
3)	LDL 70-189 + Age 40-75 + Diabetes
4)	LDL 70-189 + Age 40-75 + Calculated (Risk Factors)

INTENSITY OF STATINS		
High Intensity	Moderate Intensity	Low Intensity
Atorva 40,80	Atorva 10,20	-----------
Rosuva 20,40	Rosuva 5,10	-----------
-----------	Simva 20,40	Simva 5,10
-----------	Prava 40,80	Prava 10,20
-----------	Lova 40	Lova 20

SIDE EFFECTS		
Baseline	Routine	Sxs
Lipids	q1y	-----------
A1c	DM = q3mo	-----------
CK	-----------	Muscle Soreness (CK)
LFTs	-----------	Hepatitis (LFTs)

ACLS

RHYTHMS TO TREATMENT		
Rhythm	Drug	Electricity
VFib	Amio	Shock
VTach	Amio	Shock
Torsades	Mag	Shock
SVT	Adenosine	Shock
1° Block	Atropine	Pace
2° Type 1	Atropine	Pace
2° Type 2		Pace
3° Block		Pace

CODES	
No pulse	CPR
Shock delivered	CPR
Anything	CPR
All codes	Epi
VT/VF Codes	Epi, Amio
PEA, Asystole	Epi

AFIB WITH RVR	
Path:	Underlying stressor Ischemia, Infection, Structural heart
Pt:	Palpitations, Asymptomatic
Dx:	ECG
Tx:	NO HEART FAILURE: BB or CCB HEART FAILURE: Dig, Amio Shock: Shock

AFIB	
Path:	PIRATES mnemonic Ischemia, Infection, Structural heart
Pt:	Palpitations, Asymptomatic
Dx:	ECG
Tx:	Rate control = Rhythm Control (AFFIRM) Rhythm: Cardioversion after TTE, TEE, one month of anticoagulation Rate: BB, CCB Rate: Anticoagulate with CHADS2 **C** CHF **H** HTN **A** Age > 75 **D** Diabetes **S** Stroke **S** Stroke Score 0—Aspirin Score 1—Rivaroxaban, Apixaban Score 2+ —Warfarin or -axabans

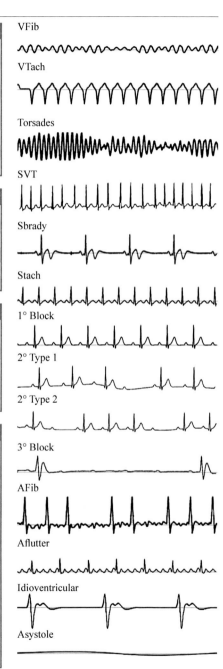

VFib

VTach

Torsades

SVT

Sbrady

Stach

1° Block

2° Type 1

2° Type 2

3° Block

AFib

Aflutter

Idioventricular

Asystole

Syncope

VASOVAGAL	
Path:	1. Visceral Stimulation: Micturition, Coughing, Sneezing 2. Carotid Stimulation: turning head, tight ties, boxer blow 3. Psychogenic: Sight of blood Cardioinhibitory surge = hypotension, bradycardia
Pt:	Prodrome (they know it's coming) One of the pathologies above Situational Syncope
Dx:	Tilt-Table
Tx:	β-blockers

ORTHOSTATIC	
Path:	1. Volume Down = Dehydration, Diarrhea, Diuresis, Hemorrhage 2. Autonomic Nervous System = Age, diabetes, Shy-Drager (Parkinson)
Pt:	Orthostatic
Dx:	Orthostatics
Tx:	Rehydrate / Transfuse Steroids if that fails Cautious standing in elderly

MECHANICAL CARDIAC	
Path:	Valvular or structural lesion = HOCM, saddle embolus, aortic stenosis, left atrial Myxoma
Pt:	Exertional Syncope
Dx:	Echo
Tx:	Treat the underlying mechanical disease

ARRHYTHMIA	
Path:	Arrhythmia, too fast or too slow
Pt:	Sudden onset, no prodrome, just happens
Dx:	ECG (usually negative) Holter (24 hour ECG) Event recorder (wear it for a month)
Tx:	AICD or Arrhythmia Meds

NEUROGENIC	
Path:	Poor perfusion to the brain (posterior circulation)
Pt:	Sudden onset, no prodrome (like arrhythmia) Focal Neurologic Deficit
Dx:	CT angiogram
Tx:	Medically manage Stenting

Asthma

ASTHMA	
Path:	Reversible Inflammation and Bronchoconstriction
Pt:	Shortness of breath Wheezing Hyperresonant Prolonged Expiration Exposure to trigger (cold air, allergens) *CBC = Eosinophilia, "Nasal Polyps"*

Dx:	Pulmonary function tests
	  - FEV1 / FVC ↓
	    - Reversible with bronchodilators
	    - Inducible with Methacholine
	Skin Test = identify triggers

Tx:	β-agonists
	  - Short-acting
	  - Long-acting (never alone)
	Steroids
	  - Inhaled corticosteroids
	  - Oral prednisone
	Stabilizers
	  - Nedocromil, cromolyn
	  - Leukotriene antagonists

F/u:	Avoid Triggers

ASTHMA EXACERBATION	
Path:	Exposure to trigger
Pt:	Exposure to trigger = wheezing, dyspnea, prolonged exhalation CBC = Eosinophilia Nasal Polyps
Dx:	Clinical X-ray (done to rule out something else) Peak-Flow PFTs (not for an exacerbation)
Tx:	IV Methylprednisolone Albuterol + Ipratroprium Steroid Taper
F/u:	Racemic Epinephrine Magnesium "stops wheezing" or "CO_2 rising" → intubate

CHRONIC ASTHMA TREATMENT	
I	SABA
II	SABA + ICS LTA = ICS
III	SABA + ICS + LABA
IV	SABA + ↑ ICS + LABA
Ref.	Oral Prednisone

ASTHMA DRUGS	
SABA	Albuterol
LABA	Formoterol, Salmeterol
ICS	Beclomethasone, Budesonide, Fluticasone, Mometasone
LTA	Montelukast, Zafirlukast
Steroids	Prednisone (oral)

Lung Cancer

LUNG CANCER	
Path:	Smoking, Toxic Exposure
Pt:	Weight Loss, Hemoptysis, Dyspnea Pleural Effusion (tap effusion first)

Dx:	1st: CXR
	Then: CT scan
	Best: Biopsy
	    - Percutaneous if peripheral
	    - Endoscopic Ultrasound if
	        proximal
	    - VATS if in the middle
	    - Lobectomy ok too

Tx:	Diagnose, Stage PFTs (can they tolerate surgery?) Surgery vs. Chemo

F/u:	Annual low-dose CT scan . . . cancer
	   screen
	    - Smoker within 15 years
	    - 55-80 years old
	    - > 30 pack year history

CARCINOID TUMOR	
Path:	Serotonin
Pt:	Wheezing, Flushing, Diarrhea
Dx:	5-HIAA in the urine
Tx:	Resection

SMALL CELL LUNG CANCER	
Path:	Smoking

Pt:	Sentral Mass
	Paraneoplastic Syndromes
	    - SIADH = HypoNa
	    - ACTH = Cushing's

Dx:	Bronch / EUS
Tx:	Chemo

SQUAMOUS CELL LUNG CANCER	
Path:	Smoking
Pt:	Sentral Mass Paraneoplastic Syndromes - PTH-rp = HyperCa
Dx:	Bronch / EUS
Tx:	Resection Chemo, Radiation

ADENOCARCINOMA	
Path:	Asbestosis cancer NON smokers get
Pt:	Peripheral mass Pleural Plaques
Dx:	Percutaneous Biopsy
Tx:	Chemo / Rads

Pleural Effusion

PLEURAL EFFUSION	

Path:	Transudate: "*Fluid*"
	   - ↑ Hydrostatic = CHF
	   - ↓ Oncotic = Cirrhosis, Nephrosis
	Exudate: "*Stuff*"
	   - ↑ Permeability = TB, Cancer,
	       PNA

Pt:	Exertional Dyspnea, Orthopnea Incidentally found on X-ray

Dx:	1st: CXR
	Then: Decubitus CXR (or ultrasound)
	Then: Thoracentesis (not loculated)
	    OR
	        Thoracostomy (loculated)
	    OR
	        Thoracotomy (empyema)
	Best: Biopsy, Gram Stain, Cytology

Tx:	If CHF, do NOT tap, just diuresis If no CHF, tap, then treat accordingly to the underlying diagnosis

THORAPROCEDURES	
Thoracentesis	Needle in the chest
Thoracostomy	Chest tube in the chest
Thoracotomy	Hole cut in the chest

LIGHT'S CRITERIA	
LDH	> 200
LDH$_{fluid}$: LDH$_{serum}$	> 0.6
TP$_{fluid}$: TP$_{serum}$	> 0.5
Any **one** signifies an exudate	

FLUID WORKUP	
Cell Count with diff	Infection
Gram Stain	Infection
Culture	Infection
AFB smear	TB
Adenosine Deaminase	TB
Cytology	Cancer
TP	Light's
LDH	Light's
RBC	Hemothorax
Amylase	Chylothorax
pH, Glucose	Other

DVT PE

DEEP VEIN THROMBOSIS	
Path:	Virchow's triad - Endothelial Injury - Venous Stasis - Hypercoagulability
Pt:	Unilateral leg swollen than the other > 2 cm Pain, Erythema, Swelling ~~Hammond's Sign~~
Dx:	Ultrasound
Tx:	Anticoagulation (LMWH → Warfarin)
F/u:	INR 2-3

PULMONARY EMBOLISM	
Path:	DVT embolizes to lung
Pt:	Wedge infarct = hemoptysis, dyspnea Pulmonary Hypertension = Heart strain Ischemia = Pleuritic Chest pain V/Q Mismatch = Hypoxemia and Dyspnea Tachycardia, Tachypnea, Hypoxia, Hypocapnia
Dx:	1st: D-Dimer rules out disease (clinic) Best: Spiral CT (CT Chest IV Contrast) Alt: V/Q Scan if Creatinine compromised
Tx:	IVF, O_2, Anticoagulation - Heparin to Warfarin bridge - 5 day LMWH or therapeutic INR 2-3, whichever is longer - tPA if massive - IVC filter ONLY if anticoagula- tion is contraindicated
F/u:	ABG: Low O_2, Low CO_2, high pH ECG: S1Q3T3 CXR: Negative Well's Criteria

WELLS' CRITERIA—CALCULATING THE SCORE	
ZOMFG I DONT KNOW	3
DVT	3
HR > 100	1.5
Immobilization (Leg Fx, Travel)	1.5
Surgery w/i 4 weeks	1.5
h/o DVT or PE	1.5
Hemoptysis	1
Malignancy	1

V/Q AND D-DIMER INTERPRETATION		
Score < 2 Low Prob D-Dimer, VQ OK	Score 2-6 Med Prob V/Q Useless	Score > 6 High Prob V/Q OK

DO I DO A CT SCAN?	
Score ≤ 4 Don't do it	Score > 4 Do it

COPD

COPD	
Time:	Emphysema and Bronchitis Genetics and Smoking
Pt:	Pink Puffer = emphysema = trapped air - Hyperresonant - ↑ AP diameter, Flattened Diaphragm - Pursed Lips, Prolonged Expiration - CO_2 retainer Blue Bloater = Bronchitis = Hypoxia - Cyanotic - Pulmonary HTN - Right Heart Failure - Hepatosplenomegaly - Peripheral Edema
Dx:	PFTS: ↓ FEV1 / FVC . . . irreversible CXR can show flattened diaphragms
Tx:	**C**orticosteroids = ICS → Oral Prednisone **O**xygen = PaO_2 < 55 or SpO_2 < 88% **P**revention = smoking cessation, vaccines **D**ilators = Bronchodilators, Ipratropium **E**xperimental = don't worry about it **R**ehab = Exercise capacity increases

ESCALATION OF THERAPY FOR COPD
SABA
SABA + Tiotropium
SABA + Tiotropium + LABA
SABA + Tiotropium + LABA/ICS
SABA + Tiotropium + LABA/ICS + PDE-4-i
. . . Add oral steroids

COPD EXACERBATION	
Path:	Infectious (viral or bacterial)
Pt:	Cough, Shortness of breath, Productive sputum Wheezing CO_2 retention
Dx:	1st: CXR (rule out pneumonia) ABG = CO_2 retention
Tx:	CO_2 = Bipap Albuterol and Ipratropium Oral or IV Steroids Abx = Doxycycline or Azithromycin
F/u:	Intubate if CO_2 rises

ARDS

ARDS	
Path:	Non-cardiogenic pulmonary edema
Pt:	TRALI, Gram Neg Rods, Near-Drowning Bilateral fluffy infiltrates on CXR Pulmonary edema
Dx:	ARDS Criteria - P/F ratio < 200 - Echo, BNP, PCWP normal - Pulmonary Edema
Tx:	Intubation PEEP Low Tv . . . 6cc/kg ideal Body weight Oxygenation Paralysis
F/u:	Fix the underlying disease

CHF vs. ARDS		
ARDS		CHF
↓	PCWP	↑
↑	LV Fxn	↓
Fluffy	CXR	Fluffy
Normal	2D Echo	LV dysfunction
↓	BNP	↑

Diffuse Parenchymal Lung Disease

DIFFUSE PARENCHYMAL LUNG DISEASE (DPLD) FORMERLY INTERSTITIAL LUNG DISEASE (ILD)	
Path:	Variable: See above
Pt:	Chronic, Insidious Onset Dry Cough Hypoxemia Restrictive picture Dry Crackles
Dx:	Chest X-ray High Resolution CT Bx = VATS
Tx:	Anti-Inflammatories - DMARDs - Biologics - Steroids
F/u:	O_2 supplementation if $SpO_2 < 88\%$

SARCOID	
Path:	Autoimmune, Infiltrating disease
Pt:	Young, African American Woman Bilateral Hilar Lymphadenopathy E-Nodosum
Dx:	1st: CXR = B Hilar Lymph Then: PFTs = restrictive disease Best: Biopsy = Noncaseating Granuloma
Tx:	Prednisone
F/u:	~~Aldolase~~ ~~ACE-Level~~
Other:	Hypercalcemia . . . VIT D from Granuloma Bradycardia / Block = infiltrating heart Restrictive Cardiomyopathy

ASBESTOSIS	
Path:	Inhaled, non-degradable material
Pt:	Construction worker Shipyard industry Lung cancer or interstitial lung disease
Dx:	1st: CXR = Pleural Plaques Best: Biopsy = Barbell Bodies
Tx:	Smoking Cessation
F/u:	High risk for adenocarcinoma of lung

OCCUPATIONAL EXPOSURES	
Pneumoconiosis	Heavy metal, ground-glass opacities
Asbestosis	Ship yards, construction, demolition Pleural plaque
Silicosis	Rock dust, sand blasting
Coal Miner's	Coal Caplan Syndrome
Hypersensitivity Pneumonitis	Noncaseating granulomas Pigeon Feathers Actinomyces

SPECIAL CONSIDERATIONS		
Exposure	*Disease*	*Correlation*
Shipyards	Asbestosis	Cancer
Construction	Asbestosis	Cancer
Aeronautics	Berylliosis	
Nuclear	Berylliosis	
Sand Blasting	Silicosis	TB
Rock Quarries	Silicosis	TB
Birds	HE	Get away from birds
Work only	HE	Get away from work

Gallbladder Disease

CHOLELITHIASIS	
Path:	Cholesterol: Fat Female Forty Fertile, and Native Americans Pigmented: Hemolysis, African Americans
Pt:	Colicky RUQ radiates to the shoulder, worse with fatty foods
Dx:	RUQ U/S = Gallstones
Tx:	Cholecystectomy (elective) Ursodeoxycholic Acid (nonsurgical)

CHOLECYSTITIS	
Path:	Gallstones in cystic ducts 1. Pericholecystic fluid 2. Thickened Wall 3. Gallstones
Pt:	Constant RUQ pain + Murphy's Sign + Inflammation (↑ Fever, ↑ WBC)
Dx:	RUQ U/S = cholecystitis HIDA scan if equivocal
Tx:	NPO, IVF + IV Abx Cholecystectomy (urgent) Cholecystostomy (poor surgical)

CHOLEDOCOLITHIASIS	
Path:	Gall Stones in Common Bile Duct ± Pancreatitis ± Hepatitis + Painful Jaundice
Pt:	Constant RUQ pain AND jaundice + Murphy's Sign + Inflammation (↑ Fever, ↑ WBC)
Dx:	RUQ U/S dilated CBD MRCP if uncertain

Tx:	NPO, IVF + IV Abx
	ERCP urgently . . . or
	     Cholecystectomy with
	          intraoperative cholangiogram

CHOLANGITIS	
Path:	Gall stone in CBD (as above) + Infxn—GNR, Anaerobes
Pt:	RUQ Pain Jaundice ⎤ Charcot's Triad Fever Hypotension ⎤ Reynold's AMS ⎦ Pentad
Dx:	RUQ U/S dilated bilary duct No time for - MRCP or HIDA
Tx:	NPO, IVF + IV Abx (Cipro + Metronidazole) ERCP emergently

Esophagitis

ESOPHAGITIS	
Path:	**Pill-induced** **Infectious** **Eosinophilic** **Caustic** GERD
Pt:	Odynophagia, Dysphagia
Dx:	EGD with Bx
Tx:	Dz-Specific AntiAcid (PPI, H2)

PILL-INDUCED	
Path:	Pill gets stuck NSAIDs, Abx, Bisphosphonates, HIV
Pt:	Esophagitis
Dx:	EGD with Bx
Tx:	EGD → Remove Pill Remove offending agent Time and PPI
F/u:	∅ Recumbency, Water with Pills

INFECTIOUS		
Candida	Oral Thrush	Fluconazole
HSV	Oral Lesions	Val-acyclovir
CMV	---	Val-agancyclovir
HIV	Opportunistic Infxns	HAART

EOSINOPHILIC		
Path: & Pt:	Asthma Allergies Atopy	Allergic Rxn
Dx:	EGD w Bx > 16 eos / hpf Trial PPI x 6 weeks	
Tx:	Oral Aerosolized Steroids	

CAUSTIC	
Path:	Kid (accidental ingestion) Adult (suicide attempt) Alkaline >> Acid
Pt:	Larynx → Hoarse, * Stridor * Esophagus → Drooling
Dx:	EGD with Biopsy
Tx:	Low Severity . . . Liquid Diet High Severity . . . NPO x 72 hrs EGD
F/u:	NEVER neutralize

Esophageal Disorders

ESOPHAGEAL DISORDERS	
Motility	NOT progressive, Foods AND liquids Dx: Barium, Manometry, EGD
Mechanical	Progressive, Foods THEN liquids Dx: Barium, EGD

ACHALASIA	
Path:	Motility Absent Myenteric Plexus LES Cannot Relax
Pt:	Knot / Ball of Food Stuck @ GE junction
Dx:	Barium = Bird's Beak Manometry—LES high tone EGD with biopsy r/o Cancer (pseudoachalasia)
Tx:	Botulinum (poor surgical candidate) Dilation (perforates) Myotomy (Best)
F/u:	GERD (if you take too much)

SCLERODERMA	
Path:	Motility Collagen Deposition LES Cannot Contract
Pt:	CREST Anti-centromere SS—Anti-Scl-70 Relentless GERD
Dx:	Barium = Normal Manometry = LES low tone EGD with Bx = Collagen
Tx:	PPI
F/u:	Serology

DIFFUSE ESOPHAGEAL SPASM	
Path:	Motility Random Sustained Contractions
Pt:	"Heart Attack" /// better with nitro Exacerbated by cold liquids
Dx:	r/o ACS first (trops, ecg) Barium = Corkscrew Esophagus Manometry = Random Contractions NO EGD
Tx:	CCB, Nitro

SCHATZKI RING	
Path:	Mechanical Ring @ GE Junction
Pt:	"Steak House Dysphagia" = infrequent, large caliber foods get stuck
Dx:	Barium = narrowed lumen / ring EGD with Bx = Ring
Tx:	Lysis during EGD

ESOPHAGEAL WEBS	
Path:	Mechanical Plummer-Vinson Syndrome
Pt:	Woman with dysphagia, Iron Deficiency Anemia, webs and eventually . . . Esophageal Cancer
Dx:	Barium = Webs EGD with Bx = Webs / Cancer
Tx:	EGD to Screen for cancer only Iron for iron def anemia
F/u:	DO NOT DO esophagectomy

ZENKER'S DIVERTICULUM	
Path:	Mechanical Diverticulum
Pt:	Old guy with halitosis . . . chokes while eating and regurgitates undigested food
Dx:	Barium = Pouch EGD with Bx = Visualization
Tx:	Surgical Resection (endoscopic or open)

STRICTURE	
Path:	GERD Grade IV
Pt:	GERD, Dysphagia, Weight Loss
Dx:	Barium = Symmetric EGD Bx = no cancer
Tx:	PPI, Dilation

CANCER	
Path:	Adeno = ↓ 1/3 Esoph = GERD SCC = ↑ 1/3 Esoph = Smoking, EtOH
Pt:	GERD, Dysphagia, Weight Loss
Dx:	Barium = Asymmetric EGD Bx = cancer
Tx:	Chemo/Radiation, Surgery

Peptic Ulcer Disease

PEPTIC ULCER DISEASE	

Path:	2 Locations: Gastric, Duodenal
	5 Etiologies:
	  - H. Pylori: Single
	  - NSAIDs: Multiple Shallow
	  - Malignancy: Heaped, Necrotic
	  - Curling's: Burns
	  - Cushing's: Steroids
	  - Gastrinoma

Pt:	ASX (20%) Gnawing Epigastric Pain Pain ↑ with food (gastric) Pain ↓ with food (duodenal)

Dx:	EGD with biopsy
	  - r/o Malignancy
	  - r/o H. Pylori

Tx:	** PPI *** Stop EtOH Stop NSAIDs Stop Smoking

H. PYLORI	
Path:	Infection
Pt:	Asx (85%) PUD + Dyspepsia (15%) MALToma (~1%)
Dx:	Serology = Test and Treat (once) Urea Breath Test = Initial Test Stool Antigen = Eradication EGD with Bx = Best (Histology)

Tx:	Triple Therapy
	  - Clarithromycin
	  - Amoxicillin (MTZ backup)
	  - PPI

F/u:	MALToma . . . treat H. Pylori, treat the cancer

ZOLLINGER-ELLISON (GASTRINOMA)	
Path:	Gastrinoma . . . ↓Gastric pH
Pt:	Big, virulent, refractory ulcers . . . And diarrhea

Dx:	Gastrin
	  < 250 = Normal
	  Between = Secretin Stim
	  > 1600 = Gastrinoma
	** SRS **
	CT scan

Tx:	Resection

Misc. Gastric Disorders

GERD	
Path:	Acid burns esophagus LES weakened Esophagitis

Pt:	Typical:
	  - Burning CP
	  - Worse with recumbency, spicy
	    food
	  - Better with antiacid, sitting up
	Atypical:
	  - Hoarseness, Coughing, Stridor
	  - Nocturnal Asthma

Dx:	PPI + Lifestyle x 6 weeks EGD with Bx (start here with alarm sxs) 24-hr pH monitoring ~~Manometry~~
Tx:	GERD: PPI Metaplasia: ↑ PPI Dysplasia: Local Ablation Adenocarcinoma: Resection
F/u:	Surveillance EGDs Nissen . . . more lifestyle than treatment

GASTROPARESIS	
Path:	Emptying Problem Idiopathic / Diabetes
Pt:	Chronic N/V Abd pain with eating Peripheral Neuropathy

Dx:	EGD = r/o other disease
	Nuclear Emptying Study
	  > 60% at 2hrs,
	  > 10% at 4hrs

Tx:	Avoid Opiates Blood Glucose Control Prokinetic Agents (metoclopramide, erythromycin, domperidone) Low-Fiber, Small volume diet

CYCLIC VOMITING SYNDROME	
Path:	+ THC
Pt:	Habitual Marijuana N/V in cycles (weeks)
Dx:	Clx → EGD → Emptying
Tx:	Stop THC

GASTRIC ADENOCARCINOMA	
Path:	East Asian Cuisine Nitrites
Pt:	Early Satiety, Weight loss, Obstruction
Dx:	EGD with Biopsy = Signet PETCT +/- Pan CT
Tx:	Resection and Chemo

Acute Diarrhea

EVALUATION OF DIARRHEA	
Severe	Fever ≥ 104, Blood/Pus, E-Lytes, ABx use, Duration > 3 days, Immuno↓
Step 1	C. diff
Step 2	Stool WBC and RBC
Step 3	∅ WBC, ∅ RBC → Ova + Parasites + WBC, + RBC → Colonoscopy
Step 4	C. diff → Treat

C. DIFF	
Path:	Overgrowth after recent abx use
Pt:	Watery diarrhea, smell
Dx:	~~C. diff Toxin x 3~~ C. diff NAAT ~~Colonoscopy = Pseudomembrane~~
Tx:	1st = PO MTZ = PO Vanc 2nd = PO MTZ = PO Vanc 3rd = Fidaxomicin
F/u:	Refractory: Fecal Transplant

DIARRHEA ETIOLOGY TO RISK FACTOR	
Entero	C. diff—Antibiotic Use
Toxic	ETEC—Travelers . . . Central America Vibrio cholera—3rd World, ∅ Boiling S. aureus—Proteinacious Foods B. cereus—Reheated rice Giardia—Camping, Fresh Water
Invasive	Salmonella—Raw eggs, Poultry Shigella—HUS EHEC (O157:H7)—HUS, Raw meat Campylobacter—Most common E. histolytica—HIV / AIDS

HUS / TTP	
Path:	EHEC O157:H7
Pt:	Blood, Diarrhea after meat ↑ BUN/Cr Anemia
Dx:	Smear = MAHA = Schistocytes Shiga-like toxin
Tx:	Supportive Care Plasma Exchange Transfusion

Chronic Diarrhea

	SECRETORY	OSMOTIC	INFLAMM
Stool Osm Gap	----		
Fecal WBC	----	----	+ WBC
Fecal RBC	----	----	+ RBC
Mucous	----	----	Mucous
Δ NPO	∅	+	----
Nocturnal Sxs	+	∅	----
Fecal Fat	----	** FAT **	----

VIPOMA	
Path:	VIP
Pt:	Chronic Diarrhea
Dx:	VIP
Tx:	Resection
F/u:	DON'T PICK VIPOMA

ZE (GASTRINOMA)	
Path:	Gastrinoma
Pt:	Virulent and refractory PUD Diarrhea

Dx:	Gastrin
	  < 250 = ruled out
	  Between =
	  > 1600 = ruled in
	SRS vs. CT

Tx:	Resection

CARCINOID	
Path:	Serotonin
Pt:	Right Sided heart fibrosis Flushing + Diarrhea
Dx:	5-HIAA Urine
Tx:	Resection

Malabsorption

CELIAC DISEASE	
Path:	Gluten Allergy Autoimmune—IgA
Pt:	Diarrhea, Bloating, Weight Loss Dermatitis Herpetiformis

Dx:	1st: Antibodies
	  - Ttg
	  - Endomysial
	  - ~~Gliadin~~
	EGD with Bx = Blunted Villi

Tx:	Avoid Gluten 3-4 Months
F/u:	Avoid gluten is the wrong answer for diagnosis

LACTOSE INTOLERANCE	
Path:	Age, Asians
Pt:	Carb Malabsorption
Dx:	Avoiding Dairy ~~D-Xylose Test~~
Tx:	Lactose Enzyme

WHIPPLE'S DISEASE	
Path:	T. Whipplei
Pt:	Malabsorption + Brain + Joint + Lymph

Dx:	EGD with Bx
	  - PAS-Positive
	  - Organisms

Tx:	TMP-SMX Doxycycline

ABSORPTION IN GENERAL	
Panc	Pancreas = Protein
Fat	A—Night Blind D—Osteoporosis E—Nystagmus K—Bleeding
Duod	Folate Iron Calcium + Carbs
TI	Bile Salts and B12

Diverticular Disease

DIVERTICULOSIS	
Path:	↑ Intraluminal Pressures, false pouches
Pt:	> 50 years old, ↓ Fiber, vegetables ↑ Red Meat Asx screening
Dx:	Colonoscopy ~~CT Scan~~
Tx:	Ø Tx High Fiber
F/u:	+ Fruits / Vegetables, Fiber Diet

DIVERTICULAR SPASM	
Path:	Contractions of diverticula
Pt:	Post-Prandial LLQ Abd pain relieved with BM (sounds like irritable bowel syndrome)
Dx:	Clx vs. IBD
Tx:	High-Fiber Diet

DIVERTICULAR HEMORRHAGE	
Path:	Arteriole Ruptures in dome
Pt:	Painless hematochezia, can be fatal or self-limiting
Dx:	Colonoscopy (for diverticulosis) Angiogram (for embolization)
Tx:	Embolize (severe) Self-limiting (often)

DIVERTICULITIS	
Path:	Fecalith blocks diverticula and infection grows, microperforation to abscess
Pt:	Left sided appendicitis Constant LLQ pain Fever / Leukocytosis Local Peritoneal signs
Dx:	KUB to r/o frank Perf CT with IV and PO contrast
Tx:	Mild: Liquid diet . . . po abx Severe: NPO . . . IV abx Abscess: NPO . . . IV abx + drainage Perf: Exlap with IV abx Refractory: Hemicolectomy

Colon Cancer

COLON CANCER	
Path:	Premalignant lesions = polyps > 50 years old, EtOH Smoking, ↑ BMI Processed Red Meat Inflammation (UC, Crohns, PSC)
Pt:	1. Asymptomatic Screen 2. Iron Deficiency Anemia > 50, Man 3. Change caliber of the stool with alternating bowel habits
Dx:	Colonoscopy with Biopsy - Age 50 q10 years
Tx:	Polyp—Polypectomy Stage I/II—Colectomy Stage III/IV—Chemo (FOLFOX, FOLFIRI)

PPx:	Screening 50-75 (± 85)
	  - Colonoscopy q10y
	  - Flex Sig q5y + FOBT q3y
	  - FOBT q1y
	  - FIT q1y (June '16 req)

FAMILIAL ADENOMATOUS POLYPOSIS	
Path:	APC Gene
Pt:	1000s of polyps by 20 Cancer by 40 Dead by 50
Dx:	Colonoscopy before 20
Tx:	Prophylactic Colectomy

HNPCC/LYNCH	
Path:	DNA Mismatch Repair 3 family members 2 generations 1 premature cancer
Pt:	Colon cancer
Dx:	Biopsy
Tx:	Resection
F/u:	Colorectal Endometrial Ovarian

OTHERS	
Turcot	Brain tumors and colon cancer Turcot . . . Turban on your head
Gardner	Jaw tumors and Colon Cancers
Peutz-Jeghers	Spots on the mouth, small intestinal tumors, colonic hamartomas

GI

GI Bleed

GI BLEED IN GENERAL	
UGIB	**Hematemesis**, Melena, Hematochezia
LGIB	Melena, **Hematochezia**
React	2 Large Bore IVs IVF bolus Type and Cross, Transfuse as needed IV PPI Call GI for EGD ----------------------- Octreotide (cirrhosis) Ceftriaxone (cirrhosis)

Dx:	UGIB: EGD first
	LGIB:
	    Colonoscopy
	        (no bleeding)
	    Arteriogram
	        (really fast bleeding)
	    Tagged RBC scan
	        (slow bleeding)
	    Pill-Cam (last resort)

VARICES	
Path:	Portal HTN
Pt:	Cirrhotic with GI Bleed
Dx:	EGD
Tx:	Stabilize . . . 1st: Octreotide Then: Balloon EGD: Banding Refractory: TIPS Transplant
F/u:	Ceftriaxone for SBP prophylaxis

PEPTIC ULCER DISEASE	
Path:	H. pylori; NSAIDS, Ca, others
Pt:	Dyspepsia, GI Bleed
Dx:	EGD with Bx
Tx:	PPI

MALLORY-WEISS	
Path:	Superficial tear in mucosa
Pt:	Weekend warriors, self-limiting
Dx:	EGD
Tx:	Supportive

BOERHAAVE'S	
Path:	Transmural tear in mucosa
Pt:	EtOH / Bulimics, wretching Fever, Dyspnea Air in Mediastinum
Dx:	1st: Gastrograffin Then: Barium Best: EGD EGD with Bx
Tx:	Surgery

DIEULAFOY'S LESION	
Path:	Normal Variant
Pt:	Painless abrupt bleed
Dx:	EGD
Tx:	Subtotal Gastrectomy

HEMORRHOIDS	
Path:	Internal: bleed but do not hurt External: no bleed, but do hurt
Pt:	Blood on toilet paper
Dx:	Clx
Tx:	Sitz baths → banding

DIVERTICULAR HEMORRHAGE	
Path:	Arteriole in dome of Diverticula
Pt:	> 50 years old painless BRBPR
Dx:	Colonoscopy
Tx:	Hemicolectomy

MESENTERIC ISCHEMIA	
Path:	"Gut Attack"
Pt:	Vasculopath, AFib, Pain out of Proportion (acute) h/o pain while eating, weight loss (chronic)
Dx:	Angiogram Colonoscopy
Tx:	Revascularize Resect

GI Bleed

ISCHEMIC COLITIS	
Path:	Watershed areas
Pt:	Hypotension first, then GI bleed Painful BRBPR
Dx:	Colonoscopy
Tx:	Supportive

Aortic Stenosis	AVM

Jaundice

HEMOLYSIS / HEMATOMA	
Path:	Excess bilirubin from red blood cell turnover
Pt:	Hemolysis Resolving Hematoma
Dx:	↑ Bilirubin, Indirect
Tx:	Monitor for Resolution Diagnose hemolytic disease

PAINLESS OBSTRUCTIVE JAUNDICE	
Path:	Cancer and Stricture
Pt:	Weight loss, clay colored stools, jaundice
Dx:	↑↑↑↑ Bilirubin, Direct RUQ U/S = Dilation MRCP = Lesion EUS (pancreas) ERCP (biliary)
Tx:	Resection

PAINFUL JAUNDICE	
Path:	Gallstones
Pt:	RUQ Pain, Tenderness Murphy's sign Worse on eating
Dx:	RUQ U/S Shows gallstones, dilated ducts MRCP for diagnosis ERCP for intervention
Tx:	ERCP or Intraop cholangiogram

Cirrhosis Etiologies

VIRAL HEPATITIS	
Path:	Hep B (both)—immuno ↓ Hep C (Chronic)
Pt:	IVDA = Hep C Sex = Hep B
Dx:	Hep C Ab Hep B Ab
Tx:	Direct Acting Agonists Ribavirin + IFN

WILSON'S DISEASE	
Path:	Copper depositions in basal ganglia, eyes, and liver
Pt:	Basal Ganglia = Chorea Liver = Cirrhosis Eyes = Kayser-Fleischer rings; Ceruloplasmin
Dx:	1st: Slit Lamp Then: ~~Cu~~, Ceruloplasmin, Urine Cu Best = Bx = ↑ Cu Liver
Tx:	Penicillamine Transplant
F/u:	Cirrhosis + Picture of eye = Wilsons

HEMOCHROMATOSIS	
Path:	Iron absorption, Iron overload
Pt:	Bronze Diabetes = DM, Cirrhosis, and Hyperpigmentation
Dx:	1st: Iron Studies - Ferritin > 1000 - * Transferrin > 50% - ~~Iron~~ Best: Biopsy = ↑ Fe
Tx:	Phlebotomy, Deferoxamine ~~Transplant~~

α-1 ANTI-TRYPSIN DEFICIENCY	
Path:	Above
Pt:	COPD + Cirrhosis
Dx:	Bx = PAS + Macrophages
Tx:	Transplant

PRIMARY SCLEROSING CHOLANGITIS	
Path:	Extrahepatic, goes with UC, IBD
Pt:	Men present with pruritis and jaundice, age 30-50
Dx:	~~ANCA~~ MRCP = Beads-on-a-string ERCP = Bx = Onion skin fibrosis
Tx:	~~Stent~~ Transplant Ursodeoxycholic Acid

PRIMARY BILIARY CIRRHOSIS	
Path:	Intrahepatic NO association with UC, IBD
Pt:	Women with pruritis and jaundice, 30-50 years old
Dx:	AMA Imaging = Normal Best = Biopsy
Tx:	Transplant

EtOH	
Path:	EtOH
Pt:	EtOH
Dx:	EtOH
Tx:	Stop EtOH Transplant

NASH / NAFL	
Path:	Fatty liver disease
Pt:	Cirrhotic changes and there isn't another cause you can find Obese people with "obese" limits
Dx:	1st: Ultrasound Best: Biopsy
Tx:	Transplant

Cirrhosis Complications

CIRRHOSIS	
Path:	Bridging fibrosis in regenerating islands of good liver
Pt:	Asx until advanced then . . . ↑ Bilirubin = Jaundice ↑ Bile Salts = Pruritis ↓ Factor 2,7,9,10 = Bleeding, ↑ INR ↓ Albumin = 3rd spacing fluid Portal HTN = Ascites Estrogen = Palmar Erythema, Spider Angiomata, Gynecomastia Splenomegaly = ↓ Plts
Dx:	Multiple Testing 1st: U/S = fatty liver, small Monitor = LFTs, Cr, INR Then = Triple Phase CT (HCC) Best = Transjugular Biopsy
Tx:	Irreversible once cirrhotic Stop Drinking EtOH Vaccinate Hep A + Hep B Transplant
F/u:	Screen AFP + RUQ U/S q6mo (HCC)

HEPATIC ENCEPHALOPATHY	
Path:	Ammonium
Pt:	Altered with Asterixis
Dx:	Clx ~~NH3~~
Tx:	Lactulose, Rifaximin, Zinc

VARICES	
Path:	Porto-Caval Shunt in Esophagus Portal HTN
Pt:	Asx screen vs. Vigorous GI Bleed
Dx:	EGD
Tx:	Bleeding = Banding (Ceftriaxone, Octreotide) Not bleeding = Nadolol, Propranolol Refractory = TIPS

ASCITES		
Path:	Fluid in Belly SAAG = Serum Alb - Fluid Alb	
Pt:	≥ 1.1 Portal HTN Cirrhosis Right CHF	Non < 1.1 TB Ca
Dx:	Paracentesis = Bx = SAAG	
Tx:	Furosemide Spironolactone Therapeutic Tap	< 2g Na < 2LH2O

SPONTANEOUS BACTERIAL PERITONITIS	
Path:	Spontaneous = Strep, GNR
Pt:	Asx Fever and Abd Pain
Dx:	Paracentesis > 250 Polys Culture is done, but not needed
Tx:	Ceftriaxone
F/u:	TP < 1.0 = FQ

SECONDARY BACTERIAL PERITONITIS	
Path:	Perforation of hollow viscous
Pt:	Abdominal pain, fever, cirrhosis
Dx:	Paracentesis > 250 polys ≥ 2 organisms seen
Tx:	Stop EtOH Transplant

HEPATOCELLULAR CARCINOMA	
Path:	Cirrhosis Hep B, HIV
Pt:	Asx screen
Dx:	Screen = RUQ U/S + AFP Triple Phase CT
Tx:	Resect Transplant RFA, TACE

PRIMARY BILIARY CIRRHOSIS	
Path:	Intrahepatic NO association with UC, IBD
Pt:	Women with pruritis and jaundice, 30-50 years old
Dx:	AMA Imaging = Normal Best = Biopsy
Tx:	Transplant

ETOH	
Path:	EtOH
Pt:	EtOH
Dx:	EtOH
Tx:	Stop EtOH Transplant

Acute Pancreatitis

PANCREATITIS	
Path:	EtOH (#1) Gallstones (#2) . . . Triglycerides, Drugs, ERCP
Pt:	Boring epigastric pain that radiates to the back, relief leaning forward, pain leaning back Anorexia, N/V Cullen (Umbilical Hematoma) Turner (Flank hematoma)
Dx:	Lipase > 3x ULN ~~Amylase~~ Amylase P CT scan only if equivocal ~~U/S~~ or ~~MRCP~~ (etiology only)
Tx:	NPO, IVF, Analgesia Refeed on Demand
F/u:	RUQ U/S to rule out gallstones BUN is single best mortality lab Apache II >> Ranson's Criteria

NECROTIZING PANCREATITIS	
Path:	Severe Pancreatitis Infected Pancreatitis
Pt:	Acute Pancreatitis + worsening outcome
Dx:	CT scan shows necrosis FNA = Bx required before abx
Tx:	IV Meropenem if + FNA

PSEUDOCYST	
Path:	Epithelial Lined pseudocyst After Pancreatitis
Dx:	3-7 weeks Early satiety, Abdominal Pain Bloated belly
Tx:	< 6 cm and < 6 weeks = wait > 6 cm or > 6 weeks drain

CHRONIC PANCREATITIS	
Path:	Recurrent acute pancreatitis
Pt:	Chronic Pain Exacerbations without ↑ lipase
Dx:	CT scan = calcifications
Tx:	Pain control NO SURGERY

Viral Hepatitis

HEP A	
Path:	Fecal-Oral, RNA Acute only
Pt:	Non-Immunized Acute inflammation ↑↑↑ AST, ↑↑↑ ALT Diarrhea
Dx:	IgM = Acute IgG = Immune
Tx:	Vaccinate

HEP B	
Path:	Sex > Drugs (needles) and Blood DNA
Pt:	Good Immune = Acute, Fulminant Bad Immune = Chronic, Cancer
Dx:	Below
Tx:	Vaccinate
F/u:	Hepatocellular Carcinoma Focus on Diagnosis Hep D (RNA) needs B, makes B worse

HEP C	
Path:	Blood (Needles), RNA Sex not a risk factor on its own
Pt:	Chronic Carrier Hep C Viral Load
Dx:	Hep C ab
Tx:	Direct Acting Antagonist ~~Ribavirin + Interferon~~ (no longer)
F/u:	Hepatocellular Carcinoma Focus on Diagnosis

HEP C DIAGNOSIS		
Ab -	HCV RNA +	Infection
Ab +	HCV RNA +	Infection
Ab +	HCV RNA -	Immune
Ab -	HCV RNA -	Unexposed

HEP B DIAGNOSIS	
Hep B s Ag	Infection
Hep B e Ag	Infectivity
Hep B s Ab IgM	Early Infection
Hep B s Ab IgG	Immune
Hep B c Ab	Immune, Exposed

Inflammatory Bowel Disease

CROHN'S DISEASE	
Pop	20-30 and again 50-75
Endo	Skip lesions Anywhere in GI tract
Bx	Transmural + Noncaseating granulomas
Pt:	Watery diarrhea and weight loss
Ca	No risk of cancer
Extra	Fistulas TI: ↓ B12, ↓ Fats Duod: ↓ Fe, ↓ Ca = Osteopenia
Surg	Fistulotomy Drain Abscess

Tx:	Mild: 5-ASA compounds don't work
	Mod: 6-MP, AZA . . . MTX
	Severe: TNF-I = Infliximab
	Flare:
	    r/o infxn with C Diff
	    Steroids, Cipro, Metronidazole
	    Perianal Dz, Drain Abscess

UC VS. CROHN'S	
Bloody diarrhea that should have the colon cut out as cure	Watery diarrhea that can't have surgery unless there is a fistula
Bloody diarrhea and pain predominates	Weight loss and malabsorption predominate
Cancer and needs surveillance, colectomy	No Cancer and does not need surveillance or colectomy
Surgery over DMARDs and Biologics	DMARDs and Biologics win the day

ULCERATIVE COLITIS	
Pop	20-30
Endo	Continuous Rectum but stays within colon
Bx	Superficial inflammation Crypt Abscess
Pt:	Bloody Diarrhea
Ca	↑ Risk of CRC Screening colonoscopy @8y q1y
Extra	PSC, p-ANCA
Surgery	Colectomy is curative
Tx:	Mild: 5-ASA, Mesalamine Mod: 6-MP, AZA . . . MTX Severe: Surgical Resection Flares: none

Acute Kidney Injury

TESTS TO GET	
1st:	U/A - Casts - Hints - Never definitive
Then:	Protein / Cr ratio = Nephrotic Syndrome Ultrasound = Hydro
Best:	~~Biopsy~~ (never the right answer except in Lupus nephritis)

WHAT THE URINE MEANS	
Nitrites	Infection
Leuk Esterase	Infection
RBCs	Hematuria
No RBCs but "positive blood"	Rhabdo (check myoglobin)
Eosinophils	AIN

WHAT THE URINE CASTS MEAN	
RBC Casts	Glomerulonephritis
WBC Casts	Pyelo
Muddy Brown	ATN
Waxy	CKD
Hyaline	Means nothing

POST-RENAL FAILURE	
Path:	Obstruction: Stone, Cancer, BPH, Neurogenic Bladder
Pt:	Abdominal Pain and renal failure Distended or Palpable bladder
Dx:	Foley Catheter = large residuals U/S = Hydronephrosis
Tx:	Catheter (relieves bladder outlet) Nephrostomy (relieves ureteral obstruction)

ATN	
Path:	Tubules Slough Off, They die Toxins: Contrast, Rhabdo Low Flow: Shock Kidney
Pt:	One of the above pathologies
Dx:	Urinalysis = Waxy Brown Casts
Tx:	Oliguric Phase: Dialysis Polyuric Phase: IV Fluids
PPx:	Vigorous hydration, reduce time in contact with toxin.

INDICATIONS FOR DIALYSIS AEIOU	
A	Acidosis
E	Electrolytes (Na/K)
I	Ingestion (Toxins)
O	Overload (CHF, Edema)
U	Uremia (Pericarditis)

CHRONIC KIDNEY DISEASE	
Hyperparathyroidism	Cinacalcet
Hyperphosphatemia	Sevelamer
HTN	CCB ACE-I BB Clonidine
Vit D	Ca + Vit D3
Dialysis	Hemodialysis TiW Peritoneal qHs

NEPHROTIC SYNDROME
HTN
Nephrotic Range Proteinuria
Edema
Hypercholesteremia

NEPHRITIC SYNDROME
Hematuria
HTN
Oliguria

Sodium

TREATMENT OF SODIUM			
	Mild	*Mod*	*Severe*
HypoNa	PO	IVF = NS	3% NaCl
HyperNa	PO	IVF = NS	IV = D5W
Sxs	Asx	In between	Coma Seizures

SODIUM CORRECTION
No Faster than 0.25 mEq / Hour
Except if seizing or in coma

OSMOTIC DEMYELINATION SYNDROME (CENTRAL PONTINE MYELINOLYSIS)	
Path:	Rapid Correction of Sodium
Pt:	Spastic Quadriplegic (irreversible)
Dx:	Clinical, Sodium rises too fast
Tx:	None, prevention only

WORKUP FOR SODIUM

1. Serum Osms
  - Hypertonic = EtOH, Glucose
  - Isotonic = Fats and Proteins
  - Hypotonic = Continue
2. Urine Na—surrogate for Aldosterone
3. Urine Osm—surrogate for ADH

If Hypervolemic → Give diuresis
If Hypovolemic → Give fluids

If Euvolemic →
  - TSH
  - Cortisol
  - Renal Electrolytes
  - SIADH is the diagnosis of exclusion

SIADH	
Path:	Hypothyroidism—TSH looks like ADH Lung lesions (Small cell, pneumonia) Brain Lesions Water, but not salt, is retained ↓ Tonicity
Pt:	Hyponatremia
Dx:	Diagnosis of exclusion U Na should be high (Aldo off) U Osm should be high (ADH on)
Tx:	Volume Restrict Correct underlying disorder

See endocrine for more on sodium.

Calcium

SYMPTOMATIC HYPERCALCEMIA	
Pt:	Stones, Bones, Groans, and Moans
Dx:	Calcium and Albumin
Tx:	Intravenous Fluids, Fluids, Fluids, Fluids Bisphosphonates Calcitonin adjunct ~~Furosemide~~

HYPERPARATHYROIDISM	
Path:	1°: Adenoma 2°: Early CKD, physiologic response 3°: Multiple adenomas from 2°
Pt:	Hyper Ca Pathologic fracture, ↓ Density Brown Tumors

Dx:	Calcium Labs
	  - ↑↑↑ PTH
	  - ↑ Ca
	  - ↓ P
	  - ~~Vitamin D~~
	Sestamibi Scan (Nuclear Scan)
	  - 1°: Single Adenoma
	  - 3°: Multiple Adenomas

Tx:	Parathyroidectomy

F/u:	Hypocalcemia post-op
	  - Perioral Tingling
	  - Chvostek's Sign
	  - Trousseau's Sign
	↓ Tertiary Hyperparathyroid with
	  - Calcimimetics = Cinacalcet

HYPERCALCEMIA OF MALIGNANCY—METS	
Path:	Mets cause bony destruction ↑ Ca . . . results ↓ PTH
Pt:	Malignancy and elevated calcium

Dx:	Calcium Labs
	  - ↑↑↑ Ca
	  - ↓ PTH
	  - ↑ P
	  - ↓ PTH-rp

Tx:	Treat the underlying cancer.

Calcium

HYPERCALCEMIA OF MALIGNANCY—PTH-RP	
Path:	Squamous cell Carcinoma of the lung ↑ PTH-rp results in ↑ Ca . . . results ↓ PTH
Pt:	Malignancy and elevated calcium
Dx:	Calcium Labs - ↑ PTH-Rp - ↓ PTH - ↓ P - ↑ Ca

HYPERVITAMINOSIS D	
Path:	~~↑ Ingestions (Calcium antacids)~~ Granulomatous Disease
Pt:	Hypercalcemia, chest lesion (TB, sarcoid)
Dx:	Calcium Labs - ↑ Ca - ↓ PTH - ↑ P - ↑ 1,25—Vitamin D
Tx:	Treat the granulomatous disease

HYPERCALCEMIA OF IMMOBILIZATION	
Path:	Old people in nursing homes It happens
Pt:	Old person in the nursing home Debility, bed-bound, or post-op
Dx:	↑ Ca ↓ PTH ↑ P ~~Vitamin D~~
Tx:	Mobilization

FAMILIAL HYPERCALCEMIA HYPOCALICURIA	
Path:	Higher set point of calcium
Pt:	Asymptomatic, Family history of high Ca
Dx:	Calcium Labs - ↑ Ca (11-12) - Normal PTH - Normal P - ~~Vitamin D~~ Urine Calcium ↓
Tx:	None needed

VITAMIN D LABS AND TREATMENT	
25-Vit D (D2)	Lab—Chronic Kidney Disease Med—Osteoporosis
1,25-Vit D (D3)	Lab—Granulomatous Disease Med—CKD

HYPOPARATHYROID	
Path:	Iatrogenic (thyroidectomy is an error, parathyroid is physiologic)
Pt:	Tetany, Chvostek's Sign Perioral Tingling, Trousseau's Sign
Dx:	↓ PTH ↓ Ca - P
Tx:	IV Calcium

PSEUDO-HYPO-PARATHYROID HORMONE	
Path:	PTH—insensitivity
Pt:	Asx
Dx:	↑ PTH ↓ Ca ↑ P
Tx:	Don't worry about it

VITAMIN D DEFICIENCY	
Path:	Dairy Sunshine
Pt:	Osteopenia Dexa Scan -2.0
Dx:	25-Vit D
Tx:	Ca + Vit D Vit D2 (25-Vit D) 50,000 qWeek Bisphosphonates (Osteoporosis)

CHRONIC KIDNEY DISEASE	
Path:	CKD—kidneys "can't win" because they are dead
Pt:	Frequent monitoring of electrolytes
Dx:	↑ PTH ↓ Calcium ↓ Phos
Tx:	Calcimimetics—Cinacalcet Phosphate Binders—Sevelamer Ca + VitD3

Potassium

HYPER-KALEMIA	
Path:	Hypoaldo (ACE, ARB, Spironolactone) Artifact Iatrogenic ESRD Ingestion + CKD
Pt:	Asx
Dx:	Potassium Level EKG - Peaked T-waves, Wide QRS
Tx:	If EKG Changes → Stabilize, Temporize, and Eliminate If no EKG Changes → Eliminate

TREATMENT FOR HYPER K			
Treatment	*Mechanism*	*Serum K*	*Total K*
IV Calcium	Stabilize	∅	∅
Na Bicarb D50+Insulin	Temporize	↓	∅
Kayexalate	Eliminate	↓	↓
Diuretics	Eliminate	↓	↓
Dialysis	Eliminate	↓	↓

HYPO-KALEMIA	
Path:	GI loss—Vomiting or Diarrhea Renal Loss - Hyperaldosteronism - Diuretics (Loops, Diuretics) - Large Volume Infusion
Pt:	Weakness, Paralysis, Loss of Reflexes . . .or . . . ASx
Dx:	Potassium Level EKG = U-Waves
Tx:	Replete K PO > IV 10mEq ↑ Serum K by 0.1mEq 10mEq / hr by PIV 20mEq / hr by Central line

Kidney Stones

KIDNEY STONES	
Path:	See next section
Pt:	Hematuria Colicky flank pain that radiates to groin No fever or leukocytosis
Dx:	1st: U/A Best: Non-Con CT Scan Other: U/S if pregnant KUB if tracking disease ~~IVP~~ never
Tx:	< 5mm: IVF + Analgesia < 7mm: MET (CCB, α-blocker) < 1.5 cm: Lithotripsy (proximal), Ureteroscopy (distal) > 1.5 cm: Surgery Sepsis: Nephrostomy (proximal), Stent (distal)
F/u:	Strain and analyze stone 24-hr urine for Ca, PO_4, Urate, Oxalate

TYPES OF STONE		
Types	*Radio . . .*	*Risk*
Ca Oxalate	Opaque	↑ Ca - Vit D - PTH ↑ Oxalate - ↓ Red Meat - ↑ Fruits - ↑ Vegetables - ↑ Vit C
Mg Ammonium Phosphate "Struvite"	Opaque	pH ↑ (alkalotic urine) Proteus . . . urea splitting
Uric Acid	Lucent	Gout, Tumor Lysis - Allopurinol (before) - Rasburicase (after)
Cystine	Lucent	Genetic Disorder

Cysts and Cancer

SIMPLE CYST	
Pt:	Incidental—you got another test Small ∅ Loculations ∅ Septations
Tx:	∅

COMPLEX CYST	
Pt:	Flank Mass Pyelo Pain Hematuria + Loculations + Septations
Dx:	CT scan or U/S (pregnant) Bx *(only if suspicion of cancer is low)*
Tx:	Resection

RENAL CELL CARCINOMA	
Pt:	Flank Mass, Flank Pain, Hematuria Cancer (↓ Hgb) Paraneoplastic (↑ Hgb, EPO) Hematogenous Spread of Mets
Dx:	CT scan or U/S (pregnant) ~~Bx~~ *(different than complex cyst)*
Tx:	Nephrectomy ("excisional biopsy")

AUTOSOMAL DOMINANT POLYCYSTIC KIDNEY DISEASE	
Path:	Adults, Autosomal Dominant
Pt:	Cysts → Flank Mass Infxn → Pyelo Bleed → Hematuria
Dx:	CT scan or U/S (pregnant) Bx
Tx:	Supportive → Dialysis or Transplant
F/u:	Pancreas → Pancreatitis Liver → Hepatitis Brain = Subarachnoid Hemorrhage - MRA, CTA

AUTOSOMAL RECESSIVE POLYCYSTIC KIDNEY DISEASE	
Path	Autosomal recessive Entire kidney is replaced by cysts
Pt:	Renal Failure Day 1 of life Flank Mass Anuric
Dx:	U/S Bx = Radially Oriented Cysts
Tx:	Supportive → Death Transplant

Acid Base

RESPIRATORY ACIDOSIS	
Path:	Hypoventilation
Pt:	Opiates → Pinpoint pupils, track marks Asthma / COPD → Wheezing OSA → Fat, Daytime Somnolence
Dx:	↓ pH, ↑ pCO_2
Tx:	No next step

RESPIRATORY ALKALOSIS	
Path:	Hyperventilation
Pt:	Pain, Anxiety Hypoxemia Fast respiratory rate
Dx:	↑ pH, ↓ pCO_2
Tx:	No next step

METABOLIC ALKALOSIS	
Path:	Hyperaldosteronism
Pt:	Volume Deplete (diuresis, dehydration, NG tube suction, emesis) Other (chloride non-responsive)
Dx:	↑ pH, ↑ pCO_2

Tx:	Urine Chloride
	- UCl < 10 → Fluids
	- UCl > 10
	      - HTN: RAS, Conn's
	      - ∅: Bartter, Gitelman

METABOLIC ACIDOSIS	
Path:	Gap vs. NonGap
Pt:	∅
Dx:	↓ pH, ↓ pCO_2

Tx:	Anion Gap
	    - > 12 → + Anion Gap
	        Methanol
	        Uremia
	        DKA
	        Propylene Glycol
	        Iron / Isoniazid
	        Lactic Acid
	        Ethanol
	        Salicylates
	    - < 12 → ∅ Anion Gap
	        Urine Anion Gap
	            - + → Renal Tubular
	            acidosis
	            - - → Diarrhea

RENAL

Macrocytic Anemia

FOLATE DEFICIENCY	
Path:	Leafy greens 3-6 week stores Pregnancy
Pt:	Tea + toast diet EtOH Pregnancy
Dx:	Folic acid levels decreased ↑ Homocysteine Normal Methyl Malonic Acid
Tx:	Folate, 1mg po

NON-MEGALOBLASTIC ANEMIA
Liver Disease
EtOH
Medications (AZT, HAART, 5-FU, ARA-C)

Metabolic Syndrome
  - Lesch-Nyhan
  - Hereditary Orotic Aciduria

B12 DEFICIENCY	
Path:	3-10 years storage Animal Products Neuro Symptoms
Pt:	Strict Vegan Pernicious Anemia Crohn's Disease Gastric Bypass
Dx:	B12 levels decreased ↑ Homocysteine ↑ Methyl Malonic Acid

Tx:	B12
	  - PO = Nutritional
	  - IM = Impaired Absorption

F/u:	Never choose Schilling Test
	PO Dose
	  Urine B12 + = good absorption
	  Urine B12 - = poor absorption
	Prolonged deficiency is loss of
	  DCMLS
	(proprioception, vibration)

PERNICIOUS ANEMIA	
Path:	Antibodies against parietal cells No Intrinsic factor, no B12 absorption
Pt:	Weakness, sore tongue, paresthesias
Dx:	Ab—Intrinsic Factor Ab—Anti-parietal
Tx:	IM B12 Cannot treat pernicious anemia
F/u:	Gastric cancer

Microcytic Anemia

IRON DEFICIENCY ANEMIA	
Path:	Slow Bleed Consumption of Iron Stores
Pt:	Woman = Menorrhagia Man = Colon cancer

Dx:	Iron Studies
	  - Iron ↓
	  - Ferritin ↓
	  - TIBC ↑
	Best: Bone Marrow biopsy (rarely
	  needed)

Tx:	Iron 2-6 weeks for anemia Iron 2-6 months for iron stores

ANEMIA OF CHRONIC DISEASE	
Path:	Chronic Inflammatory Disease
Pt:	Anemia

Dx:	Iron Studies
	  - Iron ↓
	  - Ferritin ↑
	  - TIBC ↓
	Best: Bone Marrow biopsy (rarely
	  needed)

Tx:	Give EPO Treat inflammatory disease

THALASSEMIA	
Path:	Genetic Mutations, Loss of genes, 4 α, 2 β
Pt:	Asx (1 α deleted) Minor (2 α deleted, 1 β deleted) Major (3 α deleted, 2 β deleted) Dead (4 α)

Dx:	- Iron normal
	  - Ferritin normal
	  - TIBC normal
	Hgb Electrophoresis

Tx:	Minor = do nothing Major = transfusion = deferoxamine

SIDEROBLASTIC	
Path:	Irreversible, B6, Cancer Reversible, Lead, EtOH, Copper, Isoniazid
Pt:	Anemia
Dx:	- Iron ↑ (done) - Ferritin normal - TIBC normal Best: Bone Marrow biopsy (ringed sideroblasts)
Tx:	Remove exposure, give back B6, try to treat cancer

HEME ONC

Normocytic Anemia

SICKLE CELL	
Path:	Autosomal Recessive, HgbSS Valine for Glutamic Acid Sickle under stress - Acidosis - Dehydration
Pt:	Emergency Acute - Acute Chest = MI, CHF - Acute Brain = CVA - Priapism Hospitalize Acute - Vaso-occlusive crisis Chronic - Asplenia - Avascular Necrosis - Osteomyelitis (See peds sickle cell)
Dx:	1st: Smear = Sickled Cells - Use 1st time and crisis Best: Hgb Electrophoresis (SC, SS) - Use 1st time only
Tx:	Hydroxyurea = ↑ HgbF, ↓ HgbSS IVF, O_2, Pain Control (hospital) Exchange Transfusion (emergency)
F/u:	Iron Overload (Deferoxamine)

G6PD DEFICIENCY	
Path:	G6PD ↓ Hypoxemic = Hemolysis
Pt:	African American Males Dapsone, TMP-SMX, Nitrofurantoin
Dx:	1st: Smear = Bite Cells, Heinz Bodies Best: G6PD levels 6-8 weeks
Tx:	Supportive Avoid Stress

HEREDITARY SPHEROCYTOSIS	
Path:	Deficiency in Spectrin, Ankrin, Pallidin
Pt:	Hemolysis, Spherocytes
Dx:	1st smear = Spherocytes Best = Osmotic Fragility
Tx:	Folate + Fe Splenectomy

PAROXYSMAL NOCTURNAL HEMOGLOBINURIA	
Path:	PIG-A deficiency
Pt:	Paroxysmal (once and a while) Nocturnal (happens at night) Hemoglobinuria (dark urine) + Abdominal Vein Thrombosis
Dx:	Flow cytometry ↓ CD55, ↓ CD59
Tx:	Biologics (Eculizumab)

WARM AUTOIMMUNE HEMOLYTIC ANEMIA	
Path:	IgG (Cancer, Drugs, Rheum)
Pt:	Hemolysis everywhere
Dx:	Coomb's test IgG
Tx:	1st Line: Steroids Recurrent: splenectomy Severe: IVIg Refractory to splenectomy: Rituximab

COLD AUOTIMMUNE HEMOLYTIC ANEMIA	
Path:	IgM (Mycoplasma, Mono)
Pt:	Hemolysis in the cold - Tips of digits - Tips of nose
Dx:	1st: Coomb's test negative for IgG
Tx:	Avoid the cold Refractory: Rituximab

MICROANGIOPATHIC HEMOLYTIC ANEMIA	
Path:	Schistocytes = MAHA
Pt:	TTP vs. DIC
Dx:	↓ Hgb (both) ↓ Plt (both) ↓ Fibrinogen (DIC) ↑ INR (DIC) ↑ Split products (DIC)
Tx:	See thrombocytopenia

Leukemia

ACUTE MYELOGENOUS LEUKEMIA	
Path:	Acute = Blasts Myelogenous = Neutrophils Leukemia = Cancer in the blood
Pt:	Acute, Age 67 Exposure: Benzene Radiation CML: Blast Crisis
Dx:	1st: Smear = Blasts BM Bx > 20% Blasts + Myeloperoxidase
Tx:	M3: Vit A (AUER RODS on bx) ØM3: Chemo

ACUTE LYMPHOCYTIC LEUKEMIA	
Path:	Acute = Blasts Lymphocytic = Leukocytes Leukemia = Cancer in the blood
Pt:	Acute, Age 7
Dx:	1st: Smear = Blasts BM Bx > 20% Blasts + cALLa and + TdT
Tx:	Chemo PPx CNS ARA-C ± radiation

CHRONIC MYELOGENOUS LEUKEMIA	
Path:	Chronic = Mature cells Myelogenous = Neutrophils Leukemia = Cancer in the blood
Pt:	Chronic, Age 47
Dx:	Diff (way more cells then should be) BM Bx = Philadelphia + t(9,22) + BCR-ABL
Tx:	Imatinib (tyrosine Kinase)
F/u:	Blast Crisis

CHRONIC LYMPHOCYTIC LEUKEMIA	
Path:	Chronic = Mature cells Lymphocytic = Lymphocytes Leukemia = Cancer in the blood
Pt:	Chronic, Age 87
Dx:	Diff (way more cells than should be) BM Bx
Tx:	> 65 + Asx = Ø > 65 + Sx = Chemo < 65 + Donor = HSCT

HEME ONC

Lymphoma

HODGKIN'S LYMPHOMA	
Path:	Contiguous spread Usually B sxs Pel-Ebstein Fevers Painful Lymphadenopathy on EtOH
Pt:	Nontender Lymphadenopathy ± B Sxs
Dx:	Excisional Biopsy FNA (insufficient) + Reed Sternberg Cells Stage = PET/CT or CT Chest/Abdo/ Pelvis
Tx:	IIA or better, radiation IIB or worse, chemo = ABVD or BEACOPP

NON-HODGKIN'S LYMPHOMA	
Path:	Hematogenous Spread Usually NO B sxs Burkitt's Starry Sky Extranodal Disease
Pt:	Nontender lymphadenopathy ± sxs
Dx:	Excisional Biopsy FNA NO Reed–Sternberg cells Stage = PET/CT or CT Chest/Abdo/ Pelvis
Tx:	IIA or better, radiation IIB or worse, chemo = CHOP-R, CNS PPx

STAGING		
Stage	# LN	Location relative to diaphragm
I	1	N/A
II	≥ 2	Same side diaphragm
III	≥ 2	Opposite side diaphragm
IV	Mets	N/A

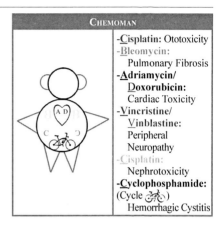

CHEMOMAN
-Cisplatin: Ototoxicity
-Bleomycin: Pulmonary Fibrosis
-Adriamycin/ Doxorubicin: Cardiac Toxicity
-Vincristine/ Vinblastine: Peripheral Neuropathy
-Cisplatin: Nephrotoxicity
-Cyclophosphamide: (Cycle 🚲) Hemorrhagic Cystitis

Plasma Cell Dyscrasia

MULTIPLE MYELOMA	

Path:	IgG
	Monoclonal expansion plasma cells
	  - Ig = recurrent infxn,
	  - Bence-Jones = AKI
	  - Osteoclasts = Lytic Lesions

Pt:	> 70s (old men)
	CRAB
	  - **H**yperCalcemia
	  - **R**enal Failure
	  - **A**nemia
	  - **B**one pain, Lytic lesions

Dx:	Spep + Upep + Skeletal Survey + BM Bx > 10% Plasma
Tx:	> 70, ∅ Donor: Chemo < 70, + Donor: HSCT

F/u:	Melphalan + Steroids
	  - Thalidomide
	  - Bortezomib

MGUS	
Path:	IgG Early Myeloma
Pt:	> 85 ∅ CRAB
Dx:	Spep + Upep – Skeletal Survey – BM Bx < 10% plasma cells
Tx:	Watch and Wait Converts to Multiple Myeloma 2% / yr

WALDENSTROM'S	
Path:	IgM
Pt:	Hyperviscosity syndrome Constitutional Symptoms
Dx:	Spep + Upep – Skeletal Survey – BM Bx > 10% Lymphoma
Tx:	Rituximab - Chemo Hyperviscosity = Plasmapheresis
F/u:	Blast Crisis

Thrombophilia

THROMBOPHILIC DISORDERS	
Factor V Leiden	Mutation
Prothrombin 20210A	Mutation
Protein C Def	Level
Protein S Def	Level
Antithrombin Def	Level

WHO GETS WARFARIN IN A DVT	
All patients	Provoked 3 months Unprovoked 6 months Recurrence lifetime
Other options	LMWH in cancer NOACs = Warfarin

DVT PROPHYLAXIS	
Risk	Trauma, Surgery (10x) LWMH PPx LMWH → Warfarin
Cancer	LMWH PPx LMWH treatment (no warfarin in met cancer)

APLA	
Path:	Lupus "Anticoagulant" Hypercoaguability in artery and veins
Pt:	Lupus + Arterial clots AND Venous clots
Dx:	Russel Viper Venom Assay
Tx:	Warfarin goal 2-3 Failure means increase INR goal

Bleeding, Thrombocytopenia

TTP	
Path:	Hyaline Clots ADAMTS-13 Deficiency
Pt:	Fever Anemia Thrombocytopenia Renal failure Neuro symptoms
Dx:	CBC ↓ Platelets Smear Schistocytes PT/PTT Normal Fibrinogen Normal D-Dimer Normal
Tx:	Exchange Transfusion
F/u:	NEVER platelets

DIC	
Path:	Fibrin Clots Tremendous catastrophic injury
Pt:	Sick as Shit Sepsis, ICU, shock, then they start bleeding
Dx:	CBC ↓ Platelets Smear Schistocytes PT/PTT ↑ Fibrinogen ↓ D-Dimer ↑

Tx:	Fix underling disease
	Give Blood products
	  - ↓ Fibrinogen . . . Cryo
	  - ↑ INR . . . FFP
	  - ↓ Plts . . . Platelets
	  - ↓ Hgb . . . Blood

HIT	
Path:	Antibodies to Platelets
Pt:	Heparin products administered 7-14 days Plts ↓↓↓ ~ 50% New Clots
Dx:	Antiplatelet Factor 4 ELISA+ Confirm with Serotonin Release Assay
Tx:	STOP HEPARIN Argatroban → Warfarin INR 2-3

ITP	
Path:	Antibodies to platelets Splenic Destruction
Pt:	Woman and Autoimmune disease ↓ Platelets
Dx:	Diagnosis of Exclusion
Tx:	Steroids IVIg Splenectomy Rituximab

VON WILLEBRAND	
Path:	Deficiency of vWD Autosomal Dominant Most common bleeding disorder
Pt:	Platelet bleed, normal count (can have Factor VIII def)
Dx:	1st: CBC = Normal Count Best: = vWF assay May have ↑ PTT from Factor VIII deficiency
Tx:	DDAVP

OTHER PLATELET BLEED NORMAL COUNT	
F/u:	Bernard-Soulier—Glycoprotein Ib Glanzmann's—Glyco IIb-IIIa Drugs—ASA, Clopidogrel, Abciximab Uremia—CKD

HEMOPHILIA	
Path:	X-linked disorder of . . . Factor 8 (Hemophilia A) Factor 9 (Hemophilia B)
Pt:	Hemarthrosis Bruises easy
Dx:	↑ PTT, can have ↑ PT or ↑ INR Mixing Studies (corrects) Factor Levels
Tx:	Factors when they bleed (short term)
F/u:	May develop inhibitors that will not correct with mixing studies

Bleeding, Thrombocytopenia

ANTIPHOSPHOLIPID ANTIBODY SYNDROME	
Path:	Lupus
Pt:	Bleeding AND clotting Hemarthrosis (bleeding) Arterial Thrombosis (clotting)
Dx:	Pt/PTT/INR Mixing Studies (does not correct) Viper Venom Assay
Tx:	Treat Lupus Heparin to Warfarin bridge for APLA

ACQUIRED FACTOR DEFICIENCY	
Path:	Liver dysfunction, Warfarin, Vit K Def
Pt:	Long ICU stay On Warfarin Has Cirrhosis
Dx:	PT/PTT/INR
Tx:	Vitamin K

Antibiotics

DIAGNOSIS TO EMPIRIC COVERAGE	
CAP	Azithromycin (PO) Ceftriaxone and Azithromycin (IV) Or Moxifloxacin (PO and IV)
HCAP	Vancomycin and Pip/Tazo (Linezolid) (Meropenem)
UTI	Amoxicillin (1st line) Nitrofurantoin (if pcn allergic) Trimethoprim-Sulfa (if no CKD) Cipro (ambulatory pyelo) Ceftriaxone (pyelo)
Skin	MRSA: Vancomycin → Clinda MSSA: Nafcillin Strep: Penicillins
GI	Ciprofloxacin + Metronidazole OR Ampicillin, Gentamycin, Metronidazole
C. diff	~~PO Metronidazole~~ Mild: PO Vanc Sev: PO Vanc + IV Metronidazole Recurrent: PO Fidaxomicin

PRINCIPLES OF ANTIBIOTIC TEST TAKING
Convenience antibiotics are almost always   wrong   - Ceftriaxone   - Moxifloxacin
The stuff the ED always uses will be wrong   - Ceftriaxone   - Vancomycin + Pip/Tazo
The test will give you a reason for why one of   these can't be used or give you an option   that has alternates

ALTERNATES	
Vanc	Linezolid
Pip/Tazo	Meropenem, Cefepime
Ceftriaxone	Ceftazidime
Cipro	Ampicillin-Gentamycin

HIV

HIV	
Path:	CXCR4 and CCR5 Receptors Gp120 RNA Virus Reverse Transcriptase
Pt:	Opportunistic Infections Acute retroviral syndrome (flu)
Dx:	3rd-gen ab test; if +, → Western blot OR 4th-gen ag-ab, confirmation built in THEN Viral Load and CD4 Count
Tx:	2+1: 2 Nucleoside reverse transcriptase-i AND 1 Non-nucleoside reverse transcriptase-i OR 1 Protease Inhibitor / ritonavir OR 1 Fusion inhibitor OR 1 Integrase Inhibitor
F/u:	CD4 climbs 50/year Viral load fall 1 log in 4 weeks

PROPHYLAXIS TO EXPOSURE	
PreP	Emtricitabine + Tenofovir
PEP	Emtricitabine + Tenofovir +/- Raltegravir
Pregnancy	AZT

OPPORTUNISTIC INFECTIONS	
PCP	CD4 < 200 Trimethoprim-sulfa (1st-line PPx) Dapsone (2nd-line PPx) Atovaquone (G6PD, Sulfa Allergy)
Toxo	CD4 < 100 Trimethoprim-Sulf
MAC	CD4 < 50 Azithromycin prophylaxis
HHV-8	Kaposi's Sarcoma Purple lesion anywhere on the skin
Candida	Oropharynx: Nystatin Swish and Spit (no systemic therapy) Esophagus: Fluconazole (systemic therapy for AIDS defining)

TB

TB	
Path:	Acid Fast Bacillus Spread through cough Caseating Granulomas
Pt:	Asx screen OR 1st exposure = pneumonia = fever + cough Reactivation = Fever, Hemoptysis, Weight Loss, Ghon's complex
Risk:	Homeless Foreign travel Prison
Dx:	Asx screen (PPD or Interferon) - PPD . . . read at 48-72 hours 5 mm immunocompromised 10 mm health-care workers 15 mm soccer moms - γ-interferon Positive or negative CXR = Cavitary Lesions, Granulomas AFB smears + Isolation
Tx:	If AFB + → RIPE If AFB - but CXR + → Isoniazid + B6 If AFB - and CXR - → Isoniazid + B6
F/u:	IGNORE BCG vaccine (pick γ-interferon if asked to choose) NEVER PPD if ever the ppd is positive If AFB positive, but weeks later it turns out to be MAC, treat as MAC

RIPE + SIDE EFFECTS	
Rifampin	Turns body fluids Red
Isoniazid (INH)	B6 Deficiency, Neuropathy Always give B6 prophylaxis
Pyrazinamide	Hyperuricemia
Ethambutol	Eye, Color Vision Disturbance

Sepsis

SIRS	
Temp	> 38 or < 36
WBC	> 12 or < 4
HR	> 90
RR	> 20

SEVERITY	
SIRS	2/4 SIRS criteria
Sepsis	SIRS with a source
Severe Sepsis	Sepsis + ↓ BP / ↑ Lactate responsive to volume
Septic Shock	Sepsis + ↓ BP / ↑ Lactate unresponsive to volume (unit, pressors)

EARLY GOAL DIRECTED THERAPY	
CVP	8-12
MAP	> 65
Uoutput	> 0.5 cc/kg/hr
SvO_2	> 70%

ACTIONS	
Antibiotics and fluids	Everyone, within 6 hours Empiric Abx 30 cc/kg IVF bolus LR = NS
Pressors	If in shock 1 = Norepinephrin 2 = Vasopressin 3 = Steroids
Lactate	Trend lactate for clearance
Oxygen	Improve oxygen delivery to tissues
Source Control	Remove plastic (lines, catheter) and drain abscesses

Brain Inflammation

MENINGITIS	
Path:	Bacterial
Pt:	Fever and a headache Stiff neck
Dx:	1st and Best: Lumbar Puncture, shows many neutrophils
Tx:	Ceftriaxone (everyone) Vancomycin (everyone) Steroids ("everyone") Ampicillin (immunocompromised)
F/u:	Syphilis: VDRL, RPR in the CSF → IV PCN Lyme: Lyme Ab in the CSF → Ceftriaxone TB: AFB positive → RIPE Cryptococcus → Crypto Antigen (not india ink) → Amphotericin RMSF: RMSF Antibody → Ceftriaxone

ENCEPHALITIS	
Path:	Viral, infection of parenchyma
Pt:	Fever and a headache Altered mental status
Dx:	1st: CT scan with antibiotics Best: Lumbar Puncture = Lymphocytes . . . get HSV PCR
Tx:	Herpes with acyclovir
F/u:	Flaccid paralysis = West Nile Temporal Lobe = Herpes Encephalitis

FAILS	
F	Focal Neurologic Deficit
A	Altered Mental Status
I	Immunocompromised
L	Lesion over the site of LP
S	Seizures
	If FAILS . . . Abx first, then CT, then LP If NOT fails . . . LP first, then abx

ABSCESS / MASS	
Path:	Mass effect
Pt:	Fever and a headache Focal Neurologic Deficit
Dx:	1st: CT scan with antibiotics If AIDS and Toxo Ag + → Treat toxo pyrimethamine-sulfadiazine and rescan If NOT aids or NOT Toxo Ag + → Biopsy
Tx:	Abscess= Antibiotics Cancer = Chemo and Radiation
F/u:	Repeat CT for toxo shows improvement, continue, if not, biopsy

Lung Infection

UTI

BRONCHITIS	
Path:	A "not that bad" pneumonia
Pt:	Fever and a cough Sputum Production
Dx:	CXR = NO consolidation (normal)
Tx:	Doxycycline, Azithromycin

PNEUMONIA	
Path:	HCAP: Dialysis, Hospitalized, Nursing home risk for MRSA and Pseudomonas CAP: No HCAP risk, usual bugs, S. Pneumo, M. Catarrhalis, H. Flu If Klebsiella, think EtOH If Mycoplasma = think Cold agglutinin disease If *Staph. aureus* = think post-viral URI If AIDS = PCP, TB, Fungus, CMV
Pt:	Fever and a cough Consolidation physical = ↑ fremitus, ↑ egophony, ↓ lung sounds, dullness
Dx:	CXR shows consolidation ~~Sputum Culture~~ Induced sputum, silver stain, for PCP
Tx:	HCAP: Vancomycin, Pip/Tazo CAP: Ceftriaxone, Azithromycin OR Moxifloxacin
F/u:	Pneumonia Vaccine (Streptococcal) Legionella = get a urine antigen

PCP PNEUMONIA	
Path:	HIV, AIDS, CD4 < 200
Pt:	Bilateral Interstitial Infiltrates Subacute Pneumonia
Dx:	Silver Stain on Sputum
Tx:	Bactrim IV Steroids if PaO_2 < 70
F/u:	Clues are ↑ LDH, but don't order it

ABSCESS	
Path:	Necrosis of the lung
Pt:	Fever and a cough Sputum Production Foul breath
Dx:	CXR= Cavitation
Tx:	Antibiotics (I&D if necessary)

ASYMPTOMATIC BACTERIURIA	
Pt:	Urinalysis for "screening" purposes and it happens to be positive
Tx:	Don't treat

ASYMPTOMATIC BACTERIURIA IN PREGNANCY	
Path:	Pregnant women
Pt:	Asx screen for pregnant women
Dx:	Urinalysis = Leuk esterase and Nitrates Urine Culture
Tx:	Amoxicillin (first-line) Nitrofurantoin (if pen-allergic)
F/u:	Rescreen

CYSTITIS	
Path:	Bladder infection = Gram Negatives
Pt:	Urgency, Frequency, Dysuria
Dx:	Urinalysis Urine Culture
Tx:	Uncomplicated: 3 days Complicated (Penis, Plastic, Procedure, or ambu Pyelo): 7 days Amoxicillin (1st-line) Nitrofurantoin (if pen-allergic) TMP-SMX (optional) ~~Cipro~~

PYELONEPHRITIS	
Path:	Infection of the kidney
Pt:	Urgency, Frequency, Dysuria Nausea, vomiting, CVA tenderness
Dx:	Urinalysis = WBC casts Urine Culture, Blood Culture
Tx:	IV abx = Ceftriaxone or Amp-Sulbact Abx x 10 days

PERINEPHRIC ABSCESS	
Path:	Walled off kidney infection
Pt:	Pyelo that does not get better
Dx:	CT scan OR ultrasound
Tx:	Incision and drainage 14 days of abx

ID

Genital Ulcers

SYPHILIS	
Path:	Treponema pallidum
Pt:	1° = Single, painless ulcer with lymphadenopathy
Dx:	2° = Rash and fever, Targetoid lesions on palms and soles 3° = Any neuro symptoms (tabes dorsalis)
Dx:	1° = Dark Field Microscopy 2° = RPR, confirm with FTA-antibodies 3° = RPR → Lumbar Puncture with CSF RPR and FTA-antibodies
Tx:	1° = PCN IM x 1 2° = PCN IM one a week x 3 weeks 3° = PCN IV x 14 days
F/u:	PCN Allergic? → Doxycycline Pregnant and PCN allergic? → PCN desensitization Jarisch-Herxheimer Rxn = fever and sxs worsen after treatment . . . give ASA

HAEMOPHILUS DUCREYI	
Path:	Gram negative
Pt:	Single, PainFUL ulcer with lymphadenopathy
Dx:	Gram stain and culture
Tx:	Azithromycin or Ciprofloxacin

HERPES SIMPLEX	
Path:	Virus that hides in dorsal root ganglion
Pt:	Painful burning prodrome
Dx:	Multiple vesicles on an erythematous base May coalesce to look like one ulcer NO lymphadenopathy
Dx:	Clinical ~~Tzanck Prep = Perinuclear halos, nuclear molding~~ HSV PCR
Tx:	Acyclovir

MOLLUSCUM CONTAGIOSUM	
Path:	Self-limiting infection
Pt:	CENTRAL UMBILICATION Multiple "vesicles"
Dx:	Clinical
Tx:	Freeze them off

LYMPHOGRANULOMA VENEREUM	
Path:	C. trachomatis
Pt:	Painless singular ulcer with painful supporative lymphadenoopathy
Dx:	Clinical . . . NAAT if prompted
Tx:	Doxycycline

Skin Infections

LICE	
Path:	Louse lives on hair-bearing regions Sharing hats, combs
Pt:	Itchy scalp Nits in hair
Dx:	Clinical
Tx:	Permethrin Shampoo

SCABIES	
Path:	Contact dermatitis from burrowing and pooping bugs / eggs Household contacts
Pt:	Itching and a rash Family members all have it Burrows between fingers and toes
Dx:	Scrape lesions, see eggs and organisms
Tx:	Permethrin Cream

FUNGAL INFECTIONS	
Path:	Fungus
Pt:	Itchy feet, groin
Dx:	Discoloration of the skin
Dx:	KOH prep = fungus Culture
Tx:	Hair or nail involved? → PO antifungals Hair or nail NOT involved → topical antifungals Terbinafine is the best

OSTEOMYELITIS	
Path:	Direct Inoculation (you can probe bone) Indirect Inoculation (hematogenous)
Pt:	Wound that probes to bone Bone Pain Cellulitis anyway (X-ray for osteo) Recurrent ulcers that do not improve or fail to heal
Dx:	1st: X-ray ~~ESR, CRP~~ Best Radiographic: MRI ~~Bone Scan~~ Best Best: Biopsy ~~Culture Drainage~~

Tx:	Surgical Debridement
	Antibiotics
	   - If not toxic, don't give any
	   - If toxic, go broad, deescalate

F/u:	ESR and CRP (track resolution, not dx)

CELLULITIS	
Path:	Bacterial infection of SubQ
Pt:	Portal = Ulcer, puncture, laceration Rash = warm, hot, tender skin with clear demarcations
Dx:	Rule out osteo . . . with X-ray Rule out osteo . . . can you probe to bone? Rule out osteo . . . but only if really concerned, with MRI ~~Culture~~ ~~Bone Scan~~ (osteo)
Tx:	S. Pneumo: 1st gen cephalosporin MRSA: Vanc IV, Clinda or TMP-SMX

GAS GANGRENE	
Path:	Dirty Wound Gas Producing Organisms Clostridium perfringens
Pt:	Cellulitis and crepitus
Dx:	1st: X-ray shows gas ~~CT or MRI~~
Tx:	EMERGENCY → Immediate debridement Antibiotics = β-lactams and Clindamycin (inhibits toxin form.)

IMPETIGO	
Path:	*Strep. pyogenes*
Pt:	Honey-colored crusts, usually on top of another wound or sore
Dx:	Clinical
Tx:	Amoxicillin If fails, 1st gen cephalosporin = cephalexin

NECROTIZING FASCIITIS	
Path:	Rapid spread of infection through fascial planes Strep Pneumo
Pt:	Rapidly expanding cellulitis Pain out of proportion with physical exam Diabetics Blue-Grey discoloration of the skin
Dx:	X-ray normal Surgical Specimen required

NECROTIZING FASCIITIS	
Tx:	Emergency surgery and debridement Broad Antibiotics Hyperbaric Oxygen

Endocarditis

MAJOR CRITERIA
Sustained Bacteremia by organism known to cause IE (Strep, Staph, HACEK)
Endocardial Evidence by Echo
New valvular regurgitation (increase or change of pre-existing not adequate)

MINOR CRITERIA
Predisposing Risk Factor (valve disease or IVDA)
Fever > 38 C
Vascular Phenomena (septic emboli arterial, pulmonary, and Janeway lesions)
Immunologic Phenomena (glomerulonephritis, Osler nodes, Roth spots, RF)

DEFINITE
Two major criteria (Blood Culture and Echo)
One major and 3 minor
5 minor

POSSIBLE
1 major and 1 minor (almost every bacteremic patient, btw)
3 minor

REJECTED
Firm alternative diagnosis explaining evidence for IE
Resolution of everything in 4 days
No pathologic evidence (a BIOPSY!?) at surgery or death
Failure to meet criteria as above

DIAGNOSTIC STEPS	
Blood cultures x 3, one hour apart, NO abx	Subacute Endocarditis
Blood cultures x 2 now, start empiric abx, follow-up cultures	Acute Endocarditis
Trans Thoracic Echo	If you aren't sure
Trans Esophageal Echo	If you are sure

Antibiotics

NATIVE VALVE	
All Native	Vancomycin

PROSTHETIC VALVE			
< 60 Days	Vanc	Gentamicin	Cefepime
60-365 days	Vanc	Gentamicin	
> 365 days	Vanc	Gentamicin	Ceftriaxone

Surgery

GO TO SURGERY IF
> 15 mm even without embolization
> 10 mm + embolization
Abscess
Valve destruction or CHF

ID

Anterior Pituitary

3 LEVELS OF FEEDBACK AND ENDOCRINE REG OF THE ANT PITUITARY				
Hypothalamus Portal Circulation	GnRH ↓	TRH ↓	CRH ↓	GHRH ↓
Pituitary Systemic Circulation	FSH/LH ↓	TSH ↓	ACTH ↓	GH ↓
Target Organ Metabolic Effect	Ovaries Estrogen Progesterone Ovulation	Thyroid T3 T4 Metabolism	Adrenals Cortisol Stress	Liver IGF-1 Growth

PROLACTINOMA	
Path:	Autonomously secreting prolactin Most common pituitary lesion
Pt:	Women: Galactorrhea, Amenorrhea, Microadenomas, No Vision Change Men: Decreased libido, Gynecomastia, Macroadenomas, Vision Changes
Dx:	1st: TSH/fT4 Then: Prolactin levels Best: MRI
Tx:	Bromocriptine or Cabergoline Surgery
F/u:	Surgery is NOT first line therapy for prolactinomas; it is for all other secreting pituitary tumors and macroadenomas

ACROMEGALY	
Path:	Growth hormone = things that can grow Child = Long bones (Gigantism) Adult = visceral organs
Pt:	Cardiomegaly → DIA heart failure Diabetes Wide-spaced teeth Hat/ring/shoe size increases Coarse features, CARPAL TUNNEL Big hands
Dx:	~~Growth Hormone~~ IGF-1 Glucose Suppression Test MRI
Tx:	Surgery first Octreotide or Cabergoline (adjunct)
F/u:	Glucose Suppression Test = give glucose, test is positive (abnormal) if the GH does not change
Wait	Carpal tunnel is more associated with RA than Acromegaly . . . don't be tricked

CUSHING'S SYNDROME	
See Adrenal	

ACUTE PAN HYPOPITUITARISM	
Path:	Infection, Infarction, Surgery, Rads
Pt:	TSH: Lethargy, Coma ACTH: Hypotension, Tachycardia GH/LH/FSH: Irrelevant
Dx:	Clinical Hormone (Cortisol and T4)
Tx:	Replace end hormones
F/u:	Sheehan's: Pregnancy, bloody delivery Apoplexy: Tumor outgrows blood supply and dies, necrosis

CHRONIC PAN HYPOPITUITARISM	
Path:	Autoimmune, Deposition, Cancer GH / FSH / LH sacrificed so that TSH and ACTH can persist
Pt:	↓ Libido, changes in menstruation ↓ Growth
Dx:	Insulin Stimulation Test - Growth Hormone fails to rise MRI
Tx:	Reverse underlying cause Replace hormones as needed

EMPTY SELLA SYNDROME	
Path:	Normal variant
Pt:	Asymptomatic
Dx:	MRI
Tx:	Reassurance

Posterior Pituitary

SIADH	
Path:	Too much ADH = too much water = patient becomes hypotonic Brain Lesion = ↑ ADH Lung Lesion = ↑ ADH (Small cell, PNA)
Pt:	Hyponatremia
Dx:	Una ↑ Uosm ↑ Sosm ↓
Tx:	Water restriction Demeclocycline Reverse Underlying disease

CENTRAL DIABETES INSIPIDUS	
Path:	Central: no ADH production
Pt:	Polydipsia Polyuria Normal Blood glucose
Dx:	Water Deprivation test - Corrects with ADH = Central DI
Tx:	Intranasal Desmopressin (DDAVP)

NEPHROGENIC DIABETES INSIPIDUS	
Path:	Dysfunctional ADH receptor
Pt:	Polydipsia Polyuria Normal blood glucose
Dx:	Water Deprivation Test - FAILS to correct
Tx:	Gentle Diuresis

PSYCHOGENIC POLYDIPSIA	
Path:	Excess free water intake causes medullary washout
Pt:	Polyuria Polydipsia Normal blood glucose
Dx:	Water Deprivation Test - Corrects with water restriction
Tx:	Stop drinking so much

ENDOCRINE

Thyroid Nodules

Test	When to Use Them
FNA	Best Test except excisional biopsy. This is the hinge point. If any doubt—get an FNA
TSH	Nodule suspected of being hot/active
RAIU	If not sure, either before or after FNA to push one way or another
U/S	Assess nodule before FNA, identify good sites for biopsy, confirm index of suspicion

Cancers	Need-to-Know
Papillary	Most common thyroid cancer, associated with XRT Orphan-Annie Nuclei and Psammoma Bodies Papillary Architecture (FNA), h/o Head and Neck Ca Positive Prognosis (Slow Growing) → Resection
Follicular	Tumor difficult to diagnose on biopsy, looks normal Spreads hematogenously, Tx resection & I2 ablation
Medullary	C-Cells producing Calcitonin = Hypo-Ca Part of MEN2a and MEN2b genetics
Anaplastic	Found in elderly patients Grows locally and quickly Dismal Px correlates to degree of Anaplasia

Men Syndromes

MEN1	
Path:	Autosomal Dominant MEN1
Pt:	Pancreas . . .Gastrinoma, Pituitary Insulinoma Parathyroid . . . Any pituitary . . . Hyper Ca

MEN2A	
Path:	RET
Pt:	Pheochromocytoma Thyroid Parathyroid

MEN2B	
Path:	RET
Pt:	Pheochromocytoma Thyroid Neuronal

Thyroid Disorders

THYROID SYMPTOMS	
Hyperthyroidism	Hypothyroidism
+ Tachycardia	+ Bradycardia
+ Diarrhea	+ Constipation
+ ↑ DTR	+ ↓ DTR
+ Heat intolerance	+ Cold intolerance
+ Weight loss	+ Weight gain
+ AFib	

GRAVE'S DISEASE	
Path:	Autoimmune disorder Thyroid Stimulating Antibodies bind to, and activate the thyroid
Pt:	Exophthalmos Pre-tibial Myxedema Hyperthyroidism
Dx:	TSH ↓ T4 ↑ RAIU: Diffuse Uptake throughout Thyroglobulin: ↑
Tx:	Medications: PTU or Methimazole Surgery: Thyroidectomy Radiation: RAIU

THYROIDITIS	
Path:	Release of preformed T4 with inflammation of the Thyroid
Pt:	Hyperthyroidism
Dx:	TSH ↓ T4 ↑ RAIU: No Uptake Thyroglobulin: ↑
Tx:	β-blockers for symptom control
F/u:	Hashimoto's, painless, then hypothyroidism De Quervain's, painful, recovery Lymphocytic, painless, recovery

MULTINODULAR GOITER / TOXIC ADENOMA	
Path:	Autonomous secretion of T4
Pt:	Hyperthyroidism Nodules
Dx:	TSH ↓ T4 ↑ RAIU: Uptake in Goiter / Adenoma only Thyroglobulin: ↑
Tx:	Resection

STRUMA OVARII / FACTITIOUS	
Path:	Struma = Ovarian production of T4 Factitious = exogenous intake
Pt:	Woman, healthcare field
Dx:	TSH ↓ T4 ↑ RAIU: NO UPTAKE Struma Ovarii—Thyroglobulin: ↑ Factitious—Thyroglobulin: ↓
Tx:	Resection Confrontation

THYROID STORM	
Path:	Excess thyroid hormone to the point of shock and life-threatening emergency
Pt:	Shock, Fever, Delirium
Dx:	T4 ↑, TSH undetectable
Tx1:	1. Propranolol (control rate) 2. PTU / Methimazole ↓ FT4 3. IV Steroids ↓ FT4 → FT3
Tx2:	Radioactive Iodine Surgery

HYPOTHYROIDISM	
Path:	Iatrogenic (most common) Hashimoto's (most common non-iatrogenic)
Pt:	Hypothyroidism
Dx:	TSH ↑ T4 ↓
Tx:	Levothyroxine
F/u:	TSH in 3 months from start, track TSH Asx + TSH < 10 = Subclinical = No treat

MYXEDEMA COMA	
Path:	Too little T4
Pt:	Shock, Freezing, Coma, pericardial effusion
Dx:	TSH ↑↑↑↑, FT4 ↓
Tx:	IV fluids (warmed) Blankets T4 IV

Adrenals

CUSHING'S SYNDROME	
Path:	Cortisol excess ACTH Dependent - Pituitary Tumor (Cushing's Disease) - Lung Tumor ACTH Independent - Exogenous Ingestion - Adrenal Tumor
Pt:	HTN, Diabetes Central Obesity / "Truncal" Obesity Moon Face Purple Striae Buffalo Hump
Dx:	1. Low-Dose Dexa Suppression test then . . . 24-hr urinary cortisol 2. ACTH 3. High-Dose Dexa Suppression test 4. MRI Brain OR CT chest / abdo / pelvis 5. Inferior Petrosal Sinus Sampling
Tx:	Resection

ADDISON'S	
Path:	Deficient Cortisol = Adrenal - TB worldwide - Autoimmune US Deficient ACTH = Pituitary
Pt:	Hypotension / orthostatics ↓ Na, ↑ K = Adrenal deficiency Hyperpigmentation = Adrenal deficiency
Dx:	1st: AM Cortisol Then: Cosyntropin Stim Test - If ↑ Cortisol → MRI - If no change Cortisol → CT abdomen
Tx:	Adrenal gland = Cortisol + Fludrocortisone Pituitary = Cortisol alone

PHEOCHROMOCYTOMA	
Path:	Catecholamine Producing Tumor
Pt:	Paroxysms Pain Palpitations Pressure Perspiration
Dx:	24 hour urinary VMA, Metanephrine CT/MRI Abd Adrenal Vein Sampling
Tx:	α-blockade β-blockade Resection

CONN'S SYNDROME = 1° HYPERALDOSTERONISM	
Path:	Primary Adrenal Tumor = 1° HyperAldo
Pt:	HTN + Hypo K
Dx:	1st: Aldo/Renin Ratio > 20 Then: Salt Suppression test Then: CT/MRI Best: Adrenal Vein Sampling
Tx:	Resection

2° HYPERALDOSTERONISM	
Path:	Young woman, Fibromuscular Dysplasia Old Man, Renal Artery Stenosis
Pt:	HTN + Hypo K
Dx:	Aldo/Renin < 10 Angiogram
Tx:	RAS: Medically Manage, no stent FMD: Stent

INCIDENTALOMA	
Path:	Asx, non-active, "thing" on the adrenal
Pt:	Asx, incidentally found on a scan for something else
Dx:	Rule out hyper-functioning adenoma 1. Renin:Aldo (Conn's) 2. Low dose dexa (Cushing's) 3. Urine VMA, Meta (Pheo)
Tx:	Ignore it, once testing is negative

Diabetes

DIAGNOSING DIABETES	

bG:	Random (needs 1)
	  ≥ 200 = Diabetes
	  < 200 = ???
	
	Fasting (needs 2)
	  ≥ 125 = Diabetes
	  100-124 = glucose intolerance
	  < 100 = Normal
	
	2 hour post-prandial glucose
	  tolerance test
	  2 hours ≥ 200 = Diabetes

A1c:	Normal < 5.7 Prediabetes 5.7-6.4 Diabetes ≥ 6.5

TYPE	NAME	MECHANISM
Sulfonyl urea	Glyburide Glipizide	↑ Insulin secretion
Biguanides	Metformin	↓ Glucose made in liver ↑ Insulin Sensitivity
Thiazolidin-ediones	Pioglitazone Rosiglitazone	↑ Insulin Sensitivity
DPP-4-i (gliptins)	Sitagliptin Saxagliptin	DPP-4-i ↑ GLP-1
GLP-1 analogs	Exenatide Liraglutide	↑ GLP-1 ↑ Incretin

DRUG	CLASS
Lantus Levemir	Long Acting Insulin
HumaLog NovoLog	Rapid acting Insulin Combo
HumuLin NovoLin	Medium acting Insulin Combo (old school, easy)
NPH	Cheap version of "Lin"
Regular	Cheap version of "Log"

EFFECT	FINDINGS
Somogyi Effect	Too MUCH insulin at night → High AM bG
Dawn Phenomena	Too LITTLE insulin at night → High AM bG
Check early AM bG to tell the difference	

DIAGNOSING DIABETES		
	DM I	DM II
Path:	Autoimmune	Path: Obesity
	∅ islet cells ∅ insulin	Insulin Insensitivity Pancreas burns out
Pt:	DKA ↑ bG ↑ Ketones ↑ Acid Polydipsia Polyphagia Polyuria, weight ↓ Onset Childhood	Pt: Obese Complications of - Diabetes - Neuropathy - Retinopathy - Nephropathy HHS = HHNK
Dx:	A1c, bG Anti-GAD ab	Dx: see to the left
Tx:	Insulin only	Tx: 2 Oral Anti-glycemics THEN insulin

PRIMARY CARE IN DIABETES	

Nephropathy	U/A → Microalbuminuria q1y
	If retinopathy & CKD,
	  presume diabetic
	  nephropathy

Retinopathy	Retina exam q1y Laser treatments
Neuropathy	Monofilament Wire to foot q1y Gabapentin, Pregabalin Soft shoes, frequent foot checks

Diabetic Emergencies

DKA	
Path:	**Type I,** Insulin Dependent DM (IDDM)
Pt:	+ Diabetic Coma + Ketones + Acidosis
Dx:	**bG 300-500** U/A: + Ketones ABG: + Acidosis BMP: + Gap
Tx:	Replete K IV Fluids—Bolus a lot IV insulin **Follow the GAP**

HHNKC / HHS	
Path:	**Type II,** Non-Insulin Dependent DM (NIDDM)
Pt:	+ Diabetic Coma - Ketones - Acidosis
Dx:	**bG 800-1000** U/A—Ketones ABG—Acidosis BMP—Gap
Tx:	Replete K IV Fluids—Bolus a lot IV Insulin Follow the symptomatic improvement

Stroke

OCCLUSIVE STROKE	
Path:	Thrombotic = Plaque → Rupture Embolic = Stroke from somewhere else (AFib, carotids, fat, air)
Pt:	Focal neurologic deficit, acute HTN, DM, Obese, Smoker, Vascular Disease (thrombotic) Young female with neck pain (dissection) AFib with valvular disease (embolic) Think FAST (Face Droop, Arm Drift, Slurred Speech, Time and transport)
Dx:	1st: CT scan (rule out bleed) Best: MRI (*tPA before MRI if acute*)
Tx:	tPA - < 3 hours if diabetic - < 4.5 hours if not diabetic - NEVER brain bleed before - No recent GI bleed - No surgery within 21 days - No trauma
Tx[2]:	Secondary Prevention Aspirin first line Aspirin + Dipyridamole if fails Aspirin Clopidogrel if Aspirin not tolerated Warfarin INR 2-3 if CHADS2 > 2 & AFib
Risk:	Statins, LDL < 70, High-potency Insulin, HgbA1c < 7 ACE-I, BP < 135 / < 85
F/u:	Echo (TTE → TEE), if clot, heparin → Warfarin U/S Carotid; > 70% stenosis or symptomatic, carotid endarterectomy . . . *must wait weeks*

HEMORRHAGIC STROKE	
Path:	Hypertension Intraparenchymal, Subarachnoid
Pt:	Focal Neurologic Deficit Worst headache of their life
Dx:	Non-con CT scan = blood
Tx:	Neurosurgery MAP < 110

BP GOALS IN STROKE (24 HOURS)	
Stroke, tPA	BP Goal < 180 / < 110
Stroke, no tPA	BP Goal < 220 / < 120
Hemorrhagic	MAP < 110

Dizziness

POSTERIOR FOSSA TUMOR	
Path:	Tumor Demyelinating Diseases
Pt:	NO Ear symptoms YES focal neurologic deficit
Dx:	MRI MRA
Tx:	Control blood flow Resect tumor

BENIGN PAROXYSMAL POSITIONAL VERTIGO	
Path:	Otolith in semicircular canal
Pt:	Recurrent and reproducible vertigo < 1 minute with head movement
Dx:	Dix-Hallpike = rotatory nystagmus
Tx:	Epley Maneuver (otolith repositioning)

LABYRINTHITIS / VESTIBULAR NEURITIS	
Path:	Post-viral syndrome, usually URI
Pt:	Weeks after URI presenting with vertigo, nausea / vomiting, tinnitus / hearing loss (loss specifically labyrinthitis)
Dx:	Clinical, diagnosis of exclusion
Tx:	Steroids but only with 72 hours of onset, otherwise, wait it out

MENIERE'S	
Path:	?
Pt:	Tinnitus, Hearing loss, episodic vertigo Lasts > 30 minutes
Dx:	Clinical
Tx:	Diuretic and Low-Salt diet

Seizure

GRAND MAL SEIZURE	
Path:	Seizure, Generalized, Complex
Pt:	Convulsions = tonic clonic jerking Loss of consciousness
Dx:	EEG
Tx:	Abort seizure = benzodiazepines

MYOCLONIC	
Path:	Seizure, Simple, Partial
Pt:	Spastic Contractions NO loss of consciousness
Dx:	EEG
Tx:	Valproate

ABSENCE	
Path:	Seizure, Partial, Complex
Pt:	Maintains tone Loses consciousness—100s of times per day Children, you think they are ADHD
Dx:	EEG
Tx:	Ethosuximide or valproate

ATONIC SEIZURE	
Path:	Seizure, Partial, Simple
Pt:	Loses tone Maintains consciousness
Dx:	EEG
Tx:	Valproate, Helmets

TRIGEMINAL NEURALGIA	
Path:	Seizure of trigeminal nerve
Pt:	Lightning pain across the face, especially while chewing or drinking cold liquids
Dx:	EEG
Tx:	Carbamazepine

STATUS EPILEPTICUS	
Path:	Sustained seizure
Pt:	Continued seizure or a failure or resolution or failure of post-ictal state for 20 minutes
Dx:	EEG
Tx:	Abort the seizure

STATUS EPILEPTICUS	
Path:	VITAMINS vs. Epilepsy (non-compliance)
Pt:	If after 20 minutes - Uninterrupted Seizure … or … - Failure to resolve post-ictal state
Dx:	If seizing, ABORT SEIZURE first EEG for seizure Check seizure medication levels VITAMINS
Tx:	For SEIZURES - Lamotrigine - Valproate - Levetiracetam For STATUS - IV Benzos, IV Benzos, IV Benzos - IV Fosphenytoin - IV Phenobarbital - IV Midazolam and Propofol

VITAMINS		
V	Vascular	Stroke, bleed
I	Infection	Encephalitis, Meningitis
T	Trauma	MVA, TBI
A	Autoimmune	Lupus, Vasculitis
M	Metabolic	Na, Ca, Mg, O_2, Glucose
I	Idiopathic	"Everybody Gets One"
N	Neoplasm	Mets vs. Primary
S	(p)Sychiatric	Faking It, Iatrogenic

Tremor

PARKINSON'S	
Path:	Loss of dopaminergic neurons in substantia Nigra, loss of excitatory signal
Pt:	Bradykinesia Cog-Wheel Rigidity Resting Tremor Gait/Postural Instability
Dx:	Clinical Best: Autopsy = Lewy Bodies
Tx:	If > 70 <u>or</u> non-functional = Levodopa-carbidopa If < 70 and functional = ropinirole, pramipexole, ~~bromocriptine~~ Add others as Levodopa-Carbidopa fails Selegiline (MAO-B) Entacapone (COMT) Deep brain Stimulation ~~Amantadine~~

HUNTINGTON'S	
Path:	Genetic, Trinucleotide repeat, anticipation
Pt:	Chorea and Dementia
Dx:	Clinical
Tx:	None

ESSENTIAL TREMOR	
Path:	Familial
Pt:	No tremor at rest, worsens with movement ♂ 40-60 yrs old
Dx:	Clinical
Tx:	Propranolol

CEREBELLAR DYSFUNCTION	
Path:	Cerebellar lesion = EtOH, CVA
Pt:	No tremor at rest Worsens with movement, gets worse with intention (closer you get, worse it gets)
Dx:	Clinical, ~~MRI~~
Tx:	None

DELIRIUM TREMENS	
Path:	Withdrawal from EtOH, Benzos
Pt:	Tremor at rest Anxiety, Hallucinating, HTN, Tachycardia
Dx:	Clinical
Tx:	Oxazepam or Chlordiazepoxide (PPx) Lorazepam prn (tx)

Headache

TENSION HEADACHE	
Path:	Muscular
Pt:	Bilateral vice-like pain Temples that radiates to neck Worsens with exercise
Dx:	Clinical
Tx:	Over-the-counter (Acetaminophen)

ANALGESIC REBOUND	
Path:	Withdrawal
Pt:	Person who takes a bunch of pain meds and then stops (even over the counter)
Dx:	Clinical
Tx:	Just get through it

CLUSTER	
Path:	Vascular Headache
Pt:	Unilateral, Lacrimation, Ptosis, Conjunctival Injection
Dx:	Clinical
Tx:	Oxygen
PPx:	Verapamil, Diltiazem
F/u:	One-time Brain Imaging (MRI > CT) scan after attacks end

MIGRAINES	
Path:	Vascular, Vasodilation
Pt:	Photophobia, Phonophobia Unilateral pounding headache Aborts with sleep, hangover the next day
Dx:	Clinical
Tx:	Mild = NSAIDs Severe = Ergots / Triptans (caution CAD)
PPx:	Propranolol best . . . verapamil / diltiazem OK

BENIGN INTRACRANIAL HYPERTENSION	
Path:	Increased Intracranial Pressure
Pt:	Female on Oral Contraceptives Headache worse in the morning Sounds like a tumor
Dx:	CT scan rules out tumor LP has elevated opening pressure, relief of pressure = relief of symptoms
Tx:	Stop OCPs
F/u:	Serial LP or VP shunt

Back Pain

CORD COMPRESSION	
Path:	Compression of the spinal cord by any means—fracture, mets, abscess
Pt:	Neurologic compromise, back pain and History of cancer Fever Urinary Symptoms Sexual Dysfunction Sensory Deficit in a dermatome Bilateral lower extremity weakness
Dx:	1st: X-ray spine Best: MRI Spine

Tx:	IV Steroids . . . then disease specific
	. . .
	   - Drain the Hematoma
	   - I&D, Antibiotics for abscess
	   - Surgery / Radiation for Tumor
	   - Surgery for Fracture

MUSCULOSKELETAL	
Path:	Muscular Strain
Pt:	Patient has belt-like pain No tenderness, No Step-offs, No Neurologic Signs < 40 years old lifting heavy weights
Dx:	Clinical
Tx:	NSAIDs and exercise ~~Rest, Bed Rest, Immobility~~

HERNIATION OF DISK	
Path:	Nucleus Pulposus
Pt:	MSK "Plus" Lightning pain that shoots down the leg with cough and hip flexion Straight legs raise elicits pain Check for plantar flexion (L5, S1) or dorsiflexion (L4, L5) Unilateral
Dx:	1st: X-ray Best: MRI
Tx:	Neurosurgery > Conservative management at 6 months The same at 1 year

OSTEOPHYTES	
Path:	Bone spurs pinch nerve at exit
Pt:	Old guy, NO heavy lifting, but sounds like herniation
Dx:	1st: X-ray Best: MRI
Tx:	Surgical Removal

COMPRESSION FRACTURE	
Path:	Osteoporosis
Pt:	Old lady with a fall, falls on her butt Pinpoint tenderness Vertebral Step-Offs
Dx:	1st: X-ray Best: MRI
Tx:	Surgery (Laminectomy)
F/u:	Dexa scan

SPINAL STENOSIS	
Path:	Canal is narrowed (idiopathic)
Pt:	Burning or lightning pain of thighs and buttocks that is worse when upright, better with leaning forward or climbing stairs Bilateral
Dx:	1st: X-ray Best: MRI
Tx:	Surgery
F/u:	Mimics claudication but has normal ABIs (pseudoclaudication)

Dementia

NORMAL PRESSURE HYDROCEPHALUS	
Path:	Normal ICP, but hydrocephalus
Pt:	Wet, Wobbly, and Weird
Dx:	CT Scan = Hydrocephalus LP = NO ↑ ICP, but improvement of sxs
Tx:	Serial LPs or VP shunt

ALZHEIMER'S	
Path:	Plaques, Tangles, Chromosome 21
Pt:	Insidious onset of progressive memory loss Short term first, then long term Sparing of social graces
Dx:	Clinical CT scan = Cortical Atrophy
Tx:	Supportive care, family education Anticholinesterase-I = Donepezil, Tacrine
F/u:	Dies from something else

PICK'S DISEASE	
Path:	Frontotemporal Degeneration
Pt:	Insidious onset of loss of personality and social graces Sparing of short term memory
Dx:	Clinical CT scan = Frontotemporal degeneration
Tx:	None, Palliative, Institutionalized

LEWY BODY	
Path:	Parkinson's
Pt:	Sort-of Parkinson's and Dementia Acute Delirium / Hallucinations
Dx:	~~Autopsy~~
Tx:	None

VASCULAR DEMENTIA	
Path:	Strokes
Pt:	Acute loss of memory or cognition in a step-wise fashion temporally associated with stroke
Dx:	CT / MRI = Strokes
Tx:	Control risk factors for stroke

CREUTZFELDT-JAKOB	
Path:	Prions, Spontaneous Mutation >> Meat
Pt:	Young, rapid dementia, myoclonus
Dx:	Autopsy
Tx:	None, Palliative

REVERSIBLE CAUSES	
List	B12 def, syphilis, HypoThyroid, CKD
Dx:	B12 level, RPR, TSH and T4, BUN/Cr, CT scan of the head, MRI of the head

Coma

COMA	
Path:	↓ cerebral function (can come back) Toxic, Metabolic
Pt:	Brain stem reflexes intact Depressed level of consciousness
Dx:	EEG (↓), Reflexes intact, EKG normal
Tx:	"Cocktail" = Naloxone, D50, Thiamine

PERSISTENT VEGETATIVE STATE	
Path:	∅ cerebral function (never coming back)
Pt:	Swallow, eat food, breathe on their own
Dx:	EEG (↓), Reflexes intact, EKG normal
Tx:	Institutionalized care . . .? peg and trache

BRAIN DEATH	
Path:	Brainstem and Cerebrum are lost
Pt:	Absent brainstem reflexes
Dx:	Two separate physicians assess brainstem reflexes and show absence Trial of breathing without ventilator
Tx:	This person is dead, withdraw care

LOCKED IN	
Path:	Pontine Stroke, Intact Cerebrum, intact heart, intact Brainstem
Pt:	Inability to move any part of their body Disconnect between brain and the body
Dx:	MRI / CTA
Tx:	Institutionalized Care

Weakness

EATON-LAMBERT	
Path:	Paraneoplastic Autoimmune Disorder Antibodies against presynaptic calcium-channels
Pt:	Proximal muscle weakness - Difficulty rising from a chair - Difficulty combing hair
Dx:	1st: Antibodies Best: EMG Then: CT Chest
Tx:	Chemo / Surgery Azathioprine

AMYOTROPHIC LATERAL SCLEROSIS	
Path:	Unknown . . . Superoxide Dismutase?
Pt:	Both upper motor neuron lesion and lower motor neuron lesions Upper = Hyperreflexia, ↑ Babinski Lower = Atrophy, Fasciculation
Dx:	r/o Spinal Lesions = XR / CT / MRI Best: EMG
Tx:	None "Riluzole" (if you see this word, it's ALS)

MULTIPLE-SCLEROSIS	
Path:	Autoimmune Demyelinating
Pt:	Neuro symptoms separated in both time and space, Optic Neuritis = ***Blurry Vision***
Dx:	1st and Best: MRI with periventricular white lesions, demyelinated plaques Lumbar puncture = Oligoclonal Banding Evoked potentials
Tx:	Acute: Methylprednisolone x 5 days Chronic: Interferon + Glatiramer, Fingolimod Symptom Control - Urinary Retention = Bethanechol - Urinary Incontinence = Amitriptyline - Spasms = Baclofen - Neuropathic = Gabapentin

MYASTHENIA-GRAVIS	
Path:	Autoimmune disease Antibodies against ACh-Receptor
Pt:	Fatigability of small muscles Blurry vision, Dysphagia worse at the end of the day
Dx:	1st: Antibodies Best: EMG Then: CT Chest = Thymic Mass
Tx:	↑ ACh with Stigmine (Neostigmine) ↓ Autoimmune - Steroids > 60, Thymectomy < 60 - IVIg = Plasmapheresis in acute Crisis
F/u:	Edrophonium not used anymore

GUILLAIN-BARRE	
Path:	Autoimmune Demyelinating
Pt:	Ascending paralysis following diarrhea or vaccination Hyporeflexia, Diaphragmatic Paralysis
Dx:	1st: Do they need intubation? . . . PFTs Then: LP = lots of protein, few cells Best: Nerve conduction
Tx:	IVIg = Plasmapheresis NEVER steroids

Approach to Joint Pain

SINGLE JOINT	VS	MULTIPLE JOINTS
Septic Crystals		Osteoarthritis, Lupus, Rheumatoid Scleroderma, Myositis, Seronegatives
ACUTE	**VS**	**CHRONIC**
Septic, Trauma, Crystal, Reactive		Osteo, Lupus, Rheumatoid, Scleroderma, Myositis, Seronegatives
ISOLATED	**VS**	**SYSTEMIC MANIFESTATIONS**
Septic Crystal		Seronegative (IBD) Lupus (Face, CNS, Renal, Heart, Lung) Rheumatoid (Nodules, Serositis) Reactive (Oral + Genital Ulcer)
DEGENERATIVE	**VS**	**INFLAMMATORY**
Osteoarthritis		Everything Else

	NORMAL	NON-INFLAMMATORY	INFLAMMATORY	SEPSIS
Appearance	Clear	Clear	Yellow, White	Opaque
WBC	< 2	< 2	> 2, < 50	> 50
Polys	< 25%	< 25%	≥ 50%	≥ 75%
Gram/Cx	-	-	-	+
Dz	None	Osteoarthritis	Everything Else	Infection

ANTIBODY	INTERPRETATION
Antinuclear Antibodies	Sensitive Lupus
Anti-Histone Antibodies	Specific Drug-Induced Lupus
Anti-ds-DNA Antibodies	Specific Lupus + Renal Involvement
Anti-Smooth Muscle Ab	Autoimmune Hepatitis
Anti-Mitochondrial Antibodies	Primary Biliary Cirrhosis
Anti-Centromere Antibodies	Scleroderma (CREST)
Anti-Ro+La Antibodies	Sjogren's
Anti-CCP Antibodies	Rheumatoid Arthritis
Anti-RF Antibodies	Rheumatoid Arthritis
Anti-Jo Antibodies	Polymyositis
Anti-Topoisomerase Antibodies	Systemic Scleroderma

Lupus

LUPUS	
Path:	Autoimmune, Complex Formation
Pt:	Women > Men Blacks > Whites
Pt:	**M**alar Rash **B**lood **D**iscoid Rash **R**enal Failure Serositis **A**NA **O**ral Ulcers **I**mmunologic **A**rthritis **N**eurology **P**hotosensitivity

Dx:	1st: ANA
	Then: ds-DNA
	  - Anti-smith
	  - Anti-Histone (drug induce)
	Lupus Nephritis
	  - U/A → Bx Kidney
	Flare
	  - Complement levels ↓ in flare
	  - Complement levels ↑ in infection

Tx:	Reduce flares: Hydroxychloroquine Control symptoms: NSAIDs Flare: Prednisone Severe: Mycophenolate Mofetil Nephritis: IV Cyclophosphamide

DRUG INDUCED LUPUS	
Path:	Drugs Procainamide α-methyl-dopa Hydralazine
Pt:	NO visceral involvement, Skin and joints only
Dx:	Anti-Histone
Tx:	Remove drug

ANTIPHOSPHOLIPID ANTIBODY (APLA) SYNDROME	
Path:	Lupus "anticoagulant" (in the lab) actually causes coagulation (in the body) Anti-cardiolipin Antibodies
Pt:	Arterial AND venous clots Lupus False + RPR . . . negative FTA-Abs
Dx:	PTT ↑, Normal INR Mixing Study Fails to correct Russell Viper Venom tests
Tx:	Warfarin + Aspirin

Rheumatoid Arthritis

RHEUMATOID ARTHRITIS	
Path:	Autoimmune Disease Women > Men Age > 40 years old Pannus Formation → Joint Destruction
Pt:	*Nobody Should Have Rheumatoid Symptoms 3 times (x)* N: Nodules S: Symmetric H: Hands R: RF or CCP S: Stiffness 3: 3 or more joints spares DIP X: X-ray shows erosions
Dx:	1st RF or CCP
Tx:	DMARDs (Everyone and early) Biologics (Severe) . . . NSAIDs (Sxs) Steroids (Flare) DMARD = Methotrexate NSAID = Ibuprofen / Meloxicam Biologics = Etanercept, Infliximab
F/u:	Screen for TB and Fungus before biologics Spine involvement = C1 and C2 Bilateral carpal tunnel could be early RA Felty Syndrome = RA + Neutropenia + Splenomegaly

Vasculitis

GIANT CELL ARTERITIS	
Path:	Multinucleated giant cells in large vessels like the temporal artery
Pt:	Age > 50 and Unitemporal head pain and tender Jaw claudication, vision losses
Dx:	Biopsy (skip, treat first)
Tx:	Give steroids before biopsy
F/u:	Elevated ESR, CRP, low-grade possible findings

POLYMYALGIA RHEUMATICA	
Path:	Similar pathology to GCA, Large-vessel vasculitis
Pt:	Symmetric pain and stiffness of neck, shoulder, and hip girdle Proximal muscle weakness but normal CK (Idio Inflam Myop)
Dx:	Clinical (normal CK, high ESR)
Tx:	Steroids
F/u:	Angiogram rules out other disease

TAKAYASU ARTERITIS	
Path:	Giant-cell arteritis of the aorta, subclavian, or axillary arteries
Pt:	Asymmetric pulselessness, discordant BPs left to right arm Pulseless disease < 40
Dx:	Angiogram (CT, MR, Direct)
Tx:	High-dose Prednisone

POLYARTERITIS NODOSA	
Path:	Medium-vessel vasculitis Hep B-related, maybe
Pt:	Infarction of multiple organs without common vascular distribution Purpura, Mesenteric Ischemia, non-glomerulonephritis, renal failure
Dx:	Angiogram = microaneurysms and stenosis
Tx:	High-dose steroids and cyclophosph

KAWASAKI DISEASE	
Path:	Medium-vessel vasculitis
Pt:	Asian child, strawberry tongue, truncal rash, palmar erythema, desquamation
Dx:	Clinical
Tx:	IVIg and ASA

CRYOGLOBULINEMIA	
Path:	Hep C, cryoglobulins Small vessel, complex deposition
Pt:	Palpable purpura, decreased complement, elevated RF
Dx:	Clx
Tx:	Steroids, Plasmapharesis

IGA VASCULITIS	
Path:	Small vessel, IgA deposition Henoch-Schonlein Purpura
Pt:	Palpable purpura, abdominal pain, abdominal bleeding
Dx:	Biopsy = leukocytoclastic vasculitis with immune complexes
Tx:	Steroids

GRANULOMATOSIS WITH POLYANGIITIS	
Path:	c-ANCA positive, small vessel, necrotizing vasculitis
Pt:	Hematuria, Hemoptysis, Sinuses
Dx:	Biopsy
Tx:	Steroids and Cyclophosphamide
F/u:	"eosinophilic" if p-ANCA, asthma, allergies and a similar presentation Polyangiitis if p-ANCA and no granulomas and similar presentation

Other Connective Tissue Dz

SCLERODERMA	
Path:	Collagen deposition disease replaces smooth muscle and skin
Pt:	Diffuse cutaneous systemic sclerosis: face, hands, feet—above elbow and knee Visceral involvement—Kidney and Interstitial lung disease
Dx:	Anti-Topoisomerase = Anti-Scl-70
Tx:	No treatment available (NO steroids—harmful)
F/u:	Renal Crisis = ACE-I Reflux = PPIs Raynaud's = CCB ILD = Cyclophosphamide

CREST	
Path:	Same as scleroderma
Pt:	Limited cutaneous systemic sclerosis C: Calcinosis R: Raynaud's E: Esophagus S: Sclerodactyly T: Telangiectasia
Dx:	Anti-Centromere Antibodies
Tx:	No treatment available
F/u:	Pulmonary hypertension without parenchymal disease

SJOGREN'S	
Path:	Lymphocytic infiltrates of exocrine glands
Pt:	Dry eyes Dry mouth Parotid swelling, dental caries
Dx:	Anti-Ro, Anti-La Schirmer Test
Tx:	Artificial tears Artificial saliva

IDIOPATHIC INFLAMMATORY MYOPATHY	
Path:	Dermatomyositis = Inflammation epimysium, skin findings Polymyositis = Inflammation perimysium, central necrosis Inclusion body myositis = Vacuoles
Pt:	Skin findings = Gottron's Papules, Heliotrope Rash, shawl sign Proximal muscle weakness (myo-pathy) And Painful tender muscles (myo-sitis)
Dx:	1st: Elevated serum CK, aldolase Then: EMG Best: Biopsy of muscle
Tx:	Cure underlying disease Steroids
F/u:	Anti-Mi, Anti-Jo, associated antibodies

Monoarticular Arthropathies

GOUT	
Path:	Monosodium Urate Crystals Increased Production → Allopurinol Decreased Elimination → Probenecid
Pt:	Podagra Single hot swollen painful joint
Dx:	Arthrocentesis Negatively Birefringent Needle Shaped Crystal

Tx:	ACUTE = Flare
	Mild = < 4 joints, digits only
	  Monotherapy
	    NSAIDs (*not if bleeding, CKD*
	    Colchicine (n*ot if chronic PPx*)
	    Steroids (*last choice of 3*)
	Mod = ≥ 4 Joints, or an non-digit joint
	  Dual Therapy
	    NSAIDs + Colchicine (preferred)
	    Steroids + Colchicine (ok)
	Severe = Same as Moderate
	
	CHRONIC Induction
	Xanthine-Oxidase-inhibitor if...
	  > 2 attacks / year
	  goal Uric Acid < 6
	Colchicine Prophylaxis until Urate <6
	(NSAIDs ok)
	
	CHRONIC Stable
	d/c Colchicine PPx after Urate < 6
	Do not stop Allopurinol in flare

F/u:	Diet: ↓ Fructose ↓ EtOH
	     ↓ Red Meat / Seafood (purines)
	
	Xanthine-Oxidase-inhibitors:
	  Febuxostat, = Allopurinol but $$$
	Urate Lowering Agents:
	  Probenecid (rarely useful)
	Intra-articular Glucocorticoids when in
	  acute flare but unsafe for all else

GONORRHEA SEPTIC JOINT	
Path:	STD → hematogenous Intracellular Organisms
Pt:	STDs, Lots of sex, no protection Urethritis, Cervicitis
Dx:	Arthrocentesis without organisms NAAT to confirm
Tx:	Ceftriaxone AND (Azithro or Doxy)

PSEUDOGOUT	
Path:	Calcium Pyrophosphate
Pt:	Single swollen joint
Dx:	Positively Bi-refringent Rhomboid shaped crystals
Tx:	NSAIDs (*1st*) Colchicine (*better as prophylaxis*) Steroids (*CKD*)

TUMOR LYSIS SYNDROME	
Path:	Large tumor burden, cell turnover Blood cancers
Pt:	Cancer getting chemo
Dx:	Renal failure, Lots of stones
Tx:	Rasburicase
PPx:	IVF and Allopurinol

STAPH SEPTIC JOINT	
Path:	Direct Inoculation (wound) Hematogenous Spread
Pt:	Penetrating trauma IVDA, Endocarditis
Dx:	Arthrocentesis with organisms
Tx:	Nafcillin . . . Vancomycin

Seronegative Arthropathies

ANKYLOSING SPONDYLITIS	
Path:	Sacroiliitis
Pt:	Low back pain Morning stiffness Better with exercise, worse with rest
Dx:	Lumbar Lateral X-ray "Bamboo Spine"
Tx:	NSAIDs (first line) Methotrexate (peripheral skeleton) Intra-articular glucocorticoids (pain) TNF-α Inhibitors (severe or refractory)

PSORIATIC ARTHRITIS	
Path:	Autoimmune

Pt:	40-50 Men
	Psoriasis + Arthritis
	"Nail Pitting," "Sausage Digits"
	An arthritis question with a picture
	   of a fingernail is Psoriatic . . . a
	   picture of a deformity is RA

Dx:	Clinical
Tx:	NSAIDs (mild arthritis) Methotrexate (moderate arthritis) TNF-α Inhibitors (MTX failure)
F/u:	Mild: < 4 joints, no erosion Mod: ≥ 4 joints, no erosion Sev: Any erosion, MTX fails

REACTIVE ARTHRITIS (REITER'S)	
Path:	STD, non-gonococcal urethritis
Pt:	Cervicitis + Arthritis Urethritis + Arthritis Urethritis + Arthritis + Conjunctivitis
Dx:	Finding the STD - Swab everywhere semen can go
Tx:	Doxy OR Azithro (chlamydia) IM Ceftriaxone (gonorrhea)

IBD-RELATED, ENTEROPATHIC ARTHRITIS	
Path:	Inflammatory, Idiopathic
Pt:	Men = Women IBD (Crohn's or Ulcerative Colitis) + arthritis
Dx:	Clinical

Tx:	Treat the enteropathy, treat the
	   arthritis
	Mild: 5-ASA
	Mod: Azathioprine or 6-MP
	Severe:
	   - UC = Resection
	   - Crohn's = Anti-TNF

Blistering Disease

PEMPHIGUS VULGARIS	
Path:	Anti-desmoglein antibodies = desmosomes Intra-epithelial lesions
Pt:	Thin, easily torn blisters (+ Nikolsky) INVOLVES mucosa AGE 30-50
Dx:	Biopsy shows tombstoning Immunofluorescence shows intra-epithelial pattern, surrounds cells
Tx:	Acute, Life-threatening = IVIG Acute, Not Life-Threatening = Steroids Chronic = Mycophenolate or Rituximab

BULLOUS PEMPHIGOID	
Path:	Anti-hemidesmosome antibody Sub-epidermal lesion
Pt:	Tense, Rigid Bullae (- Nikolsky) No mucosa AGE 70-80
Dx:	Biopsy intact epithelium detached from basement membrane Immunofluorescence shows antibodies at dermal-epidermal junction

Tx:	Steroids
	    - Topical for limited
	    - Systemic for severe
	Mild: Dapsone + Nicotinamide

DERMATITIS HERPETIFORMIS	
Path:	Deposition Disease, Papillae IgA Anti-transglutaminase Cutaneous manifestation of Celiac Sprue
Pt:	Palpable pruritis rash on extensor surfaces and buttocks
Dx:	Anti-Transglutaminase, Anti-Endomysial EGD = smooth villi Biopsy NOT needed = neutrophilic abscess
Tx:	Remove gluten from diet Temporize with dapsone

PORPHYRIA CUTANEA TARDA	
Path:	Most common porphyria Uroporphyrin Decarboxylase deficiency Accumulation of Uroporphyrins
Pt:	Bullae on sun-exposed lesions
Dx:	Coral red urine under Wood's Lamp 24-hour urine collection for uroporphyrins
Tx:	Avoid the sun
F/u:	Look for Hemochromatosis, Hep C, EtOH, and OCPs

Papulosquamous Dermatoses

SEBORRHEIC DERMATITIS	
Path:	Fungal Infection "Dandruff Plus"
Pt:	Rash and Flakes seen on Scalp and Eyebrows, hair-bearing regions only
Dx:	Clinical
Tx:	Selenium Shampoo
F/u:	HIV, Cradle Cap, Parkinson's

PSORIASIS	
Path:	Autoimmune disease, T-Helper Cells Excess Stratum Corneum
Pt:	Symmetric, well-demarcated patches with silvery scales that bleed when picked Nail Pitting, Onycholysis (nail detachment)
Dx:	Clinical (may biopsy to rule out lymphoma)
Tx:	1st UV Light Alternative: Topical Steroids (use sparingly) Flare: Oral Steroids Recalcitrant: Immune Modulators such as Tacrolimus
F/u:	Joint pain, seronegative spondyloarthropathy

PITYRIASIS ROSEA	
Path:	Benign, Self-Limiting, Idiopathic
Pt:	Flat oval-shaped salmon-colored macule (hyperpigmentation in dark skin) Scaling lesion that does not reach the border (trailing scale)
Dx:	RPR to rule out Syphilis, Pityriasis is clinical
Tx:	None, self-limiting
F/u:	If on palms and soles, syphilis likely, should normally spare palms and soles

LICHEN PLANUS	
Path:	Inflammatory, Idiopathic
Pt:	Intensely pruritic pink/purple flat-topped papules with a reticulated network of fine white lines Wrists and ankles common, can be in mouth or vagina
Dx:	Clinical
Tx:	Topical Steroids (first line) UV light (adjunct) Oral steroids (severe) Immune Modulators (recalcitrant)
F/u:	Drug induced from ACE-I, Thiazides, Loops

DERM

Eczematous Dermatoses

ATOPIC DERMATITIS (ECZEMA)	
Path:	Immune reaction to allergens or foods
Pt:	Adult: symmetrical lichenification wherever the patient can reach to scratch Child: dry, red, itchy rash on cheeks and extensor surfaces. Look for Asthma and Allergies along with Atopy.
Dx:	Clinical
Tx:	Avoidance of triggers (remove foods) Topical steroids for adult (brief use)

CONTACT DERMATITIS	
Path:	Hypersensitivity Type IV reaction Latex, Nickel, Poison Ivy
Pt:	Well demarcated red rash in the shape of an object or clothing Pruritic, raised, and red
Dx:	Clinical
Tx:	Avoid Contact with triggers Topical steroids

STASIS DERMATITIS	
Path:	Skin changes associated with edema
Pt:	Edema in an extremity, chronic Brownish discoloration, erythema, scaling at site of edema
Dx:	Clinical ~~Biopsy~~
Tx:	Get the fluid out of the extremity with either diuretics if overloaded or compression stockings / leg elevation

HAND DERMATITIS	
Path:	Dermatitis isolated to the hands in someone who washes their hands a lot or deals with chemicals
Pt:	Food-service worker, health-care worker
Dx:	Clinical
Tx:	Moisturizers and avoidance of harsh soaps

Hypersensitivity Reactions

URTICARIA	
Path:	Type I Hypersensitivity IgE induced Mast cell degranulation leading to Histamine release = leaky capillaries
Pt:	Annular, blanching red papule following any antigen exposure (bee stings, heat, pressure, medication)
Dx:	Clinical
Tx:	Antihistamine
F/u:	Send for RAST to identify culprit antigen
F/u:	If anaphylaxis (hypotension, wheezing) give SubQ Epi, followed by steroids, H1-blocker and H2-blocker. Epi is crucial, and is first.

DRUG REACTION	
Path:	Autoimmune
Pt:	Pink morbilliform rash occurring 7-14 days after drug exposure, usually in hospitalized patients If day 2-3 after a drug, that ISN'T the cause Wide-spread, symmetric, and pruritic
Dx:	Clinical
Tx:	Remove offending agent Diphenhydramine for mild symptoms Corticosteroids for severe symptoms

ERYTHEMA MULTIFORME	
Path:	Drug reaction, HSV reaction
Pt:	Targetoid lesions that appear on palms and soles
Dx:	Clinical
Tx:	Acyclovir if HSV related Self-limited otherwise
F/u:	If involving the oral mucosa, it is considered Erythema Multiforme major, and is SJS spectrum
F/u:	Syphilis can also present with Targetoid lesions on palms and soles

STEVENS–JOHNSON SYNDROME/ TOXIC EPIDERMAL NEC	
Path:	Drug reaction
Pt:	+ Nikolsky + Oral Involvement BSA: < 10% SJS > 30% TENS
Dx:	Biopsy SJS = Basal Cell Degeneration TENS = Total epidermal thickness necrosis
Tx:	Admit to burn unit, supportive care NO steroids Withdraw all medications

STAPHYLOCOCCAL SCALDED SKIN SYNDROME	
Path:	Intraepidermal lesions from Staph Toxin targeting desmoglein (desmosomes)
Pt:	NO mucosal involvement Febrile, sloughing of skin, skin folds first off the axillae and inguinal creases
Dx:	Biopsy
Tx:	Clindamycin (stop toxin production)

Hyperpigmentation

NEVUS	
Path:	Benign hyperplasia of melanocytes
Pt:	Raised, painless, pigmented lesion that has none of the ABCDE below. If hair-bearing, it is benign
Dx:	ABCDE . . . any one means malignancy - **A**symmetric - **B**order irregularity - **C**olor mixed - **D**iameter large (> 5 mm) - **E**volving over time
Tx:	Wide Excisional Biopsy if you think Melanoma. Leave it alone if all ABCDE negative.

SEBORRHEIC KERATOSIS	
Path:	Looks like cancer, but isn't
Pt:	Large, brown, greasy, "stuck on" lesions Elderly
Dx:	Clinical
Tx:	Leave it alone
F/u:	Biopsy if changing, if not changing, leave it alone. It could be cancer if it is changing.

ACTINIC KERATOSIS	
Path:	Premalignant lesion (squamous cell carcinoma in the making)
Pt:	Sun-exposed area (hands, face, back) Sun-exposed person (sailor, farmer) Erythematous with sandpaper-like yellow to brown scale
Dx:	Biopsy
Tx:	Primary Prevention is key Cryosurgery if small lesion 5-FU if diffuse

SQUAMOUS CELL CARCINOMA	
Path:	Actinic Keratosis → Carcinoma in situ → Invasive Carcinoma (DOES metastasize)
Pt:	Sun-exposed area Sun-exposed person Lesion on the lower lip Dark lesion on the face, hands, back Ulcers that fail to heal (Marjolin's ulcer)
Dx:	Biopsy
Tx:	Surgical Resection

KERATOACANTHOMAS	
Path:	Benign lesions that look like SCC
Pt:	They have SCC except it grew rapidly and then resolved spontaneously
Dx:	Surgical Resection
Tx:	Surgical Resection

KAPOSI'S SARCOMA	
Path:	Malignancy of vascular endothelial cells AIDS (CD4 < 200) and HHV-8 coinfection
Pt	Purple lesions that can be literally anywhere, mouth, arms, intestines
Tx:	HAART. Treat AIDS, this gets better
F/u:	Local or systemic chemo may be needed in refractory cases (do not learn chemo)

For Skin cancer, see Surgery Subspecialty: Skin Cancer.

Hypopigmentation

TINEA VERSICOLOR	
Path:	Infection with the fungus Malassezia furfur
Pt:	Small scaly patches of hyper and hypopigmentation
Dx:	KOH prep = Spaghetti and Meatballs, actually Hyphae and Spores
Tx:	Selenium Sulfide

VITILIGO	
Path:	Autoimmune disease
Pt:	Sharply demarcated, small patches of depigmented skin, often on face, hands and genitalia
Dx:	Wood's Lamp shows NO pigment Biopsy = absence of melanocytes

Tx:	None
	Cosmetics
	   - Bleaching to lighten uniformity
	   - Dyes/makeup to darken uniformity

ALBINISM	
Path:	Tyrosinase Deficiency
Pt:	Pale skin, pale eyes, pale hair
Dx:	Clinical
Tx:	Supportive, avoid UV light
F/u:	PKU has funny smell, Intellectual Disability, seizures in addition to pale skin and fair hair. Screened for at birth.

ASH LEAF	
Path:	Hypopigmented (NOT depigmented)
Pt:	Child, Hypopigmented
Dx:	Wood's Lamp = Ash Leaf CT scan head = Tubers
Tx:	Nothing can be done about Tuberous Sclerosis. Supportive care

DERM

Skin Infections

IMPETIGO	
Path:	Infection with *Strep. pyogenes* Infection with *Staph. aureus* (bullous)
Pt:	Child Honey-Crusted lesions on face
Dx:	Clinical
Tx:	Local disease = Mupirocin Lots of disease = Amoxicillin (Strep) Refractory = Clindamycin (Staph)
F/u:	Can cause post-strep glomerulonephritis CanNOT cause rheumatic fever

ERYSIPELAS	
Path:	Infection of strep in lymphatics

Pt:	Dark red, clearly defined lesion in
	    the shape of the lymphatics (tracks
	    or lines)

Dx:	Clinical
Tx:	β-lactams, amoxicillin (strep)

ACNE VULGARIS	
Path:	Propionibacterium acnes
Pt:	Zits. Acne.
Dx:	Clinical
Tx:	Comedones = Topical retinoids Inflamed Comedone = Topical retinoids and benzoyl peroxide Severe Pustular = Oral Abx (Doxy) Resistant disease = Isotretinoin
F/u:	UPT before Isotretinoin (teratogen)

For more details on skin and soft tissue
infections, see infectious disease.

Alopecia

ALOPECIA AREATA	
Path:	Autoimmune Disease Well defined circular bald spot
Pt:	May include entire body Exclamation-point sign
Dx:	Clinical, rule out Tinea Capitis if in question
Tx:	Steroids

TRICHOTILLOMANIA	
Path:	Compulsive disorder (OCD, PTSD, MDD)
Pt:	Patchy alopecia Hair in different lengths of growth Women
Dx:	Clinical, can use a "window"
Tx:	Treat the psychiatric disease

TINEA CAPITIS	
Path:	Fungal infection, Trichophyton tonsurans
Pt:	Well defined circular bald spot All hairs at equal length
Dx:	KOH prep, ~~Wood's Lamp~~
Tx:	Oral anti-fungals (Griseofulvin) Hair loss permanent if not treated

TRACTION ALOPECIA	
Path:	Scarring from Pulling Hair Tightly
Pt:	Tight Braiding, Pony-Tails Hair loss is preventable, but irreversible
Dx:	Clinical
Tx:	None

CHEMO	
Path:	Chemo targets rapidly dividing cells
Pt:	Patients can lose hair during chemo Clinical
Dx:	None
Tx:	None

MALE PATTERN BALDNESS	
Path:	5DHT (androgen) driven loss of hair
Pt:	Crown thins, then loses hair Rest of hair on top of head then follows
Dx:	Clinical
Tx:	1st Minoxidil topical Best Minoxidil topical and Finasteride oral Women = OCPs and Spironolactone

DERM

Newborn Management

APGAR SCORING

	0	1	2
Appearance	Blue/Pale	Acrocyanosis	Pink
Pulse	Absent	< 100	> 100
Grimace	Absent	Lots of stim	With Stim
Activity	Absent	Flexion	Resist Extension
Respiration	Absent	Irregular	Strong

NEONATAL APNEA

Primary		Secondary
Understimulation C-Section	Path:	Uncertain
No respirations from the start	Pt:	Baby was breathing then stops
Clx	Dx:	Ensure patent airway
Stimulate baby Suction	Tx:	PPV

NEONATAL DYSPNEA

TTN		RDS
Self-limiting C-sections	Path:	Developmental Deficient Surfactant
(Near)-Term Grunting	Pt:	Premature Perinatal Distress
Hyperextended Wet	Dx:	Hypoextended Atelectasis
Positive Pressure Ventilation	Tx:	Intubation and Surfactant

HYPOGLYCEMIA

Path:	Risk factors Large gestational age, infant DM mother Small gestational age, IUGR
Pt:	Jitteriness, Tremors, Lethargy, Poor Feeding
Dx:	Every baby gets a glucose check
Tx:	If Sx = IV glucose If Asx = Feed
F/u:	Sepsis

Neonatal ICU

BRONCHOPULMONARY DYSPLASIA

Path:	↓ Surfactant = RDS Prolonged damage = Scarring
Pt:	↑ O_2 Demands FiO_2 required > 28 days Lung-Protective Strats
Dx:	X-ray = Ground glass opacities
Tx:	Surfactant (post-birth) Steroids (pre-birth)
F/u:	BPD is to RDS (peds) as DPLD is to ARDS (adult)

RETINOPATHY OF PREMATURITY

Path:	Neoangiogenesis gone awry ↑ FiO_2
Pt:	Premature infant requiring O_2
Dx:	Eye exam (all premies)
Tx:	Laser
F/u:	Glaucoma

INTRAVENTRICULAR HEMORRHAGE

Path:	Highly vascular ventricles Labile pressures
Pt:	Premie . . . ASX ↑ ICP (fontanelles)
Dx:	Cranial Doppler (all premies)
Tx:	↓ ICP . . . Shunts, Drains
F/u:	Intellectual Disability, Seizures

NECROTIZING ENTEROCOLITIS

Path:	Dead Gut
Pt:	Premie . . . bloody BM
Dx:	X-ray = Pneumatosis Intestinalis
Tx:	NPO, IV Abx, TPN
F/u:	Surgery

FTPM and Constipation

IMPERFORATE ANUS	
Path:	VACTERL
Pt:	∅ Hole on inspection (± fistula) Never first temp rectally
Dx:	Visual Inspection . . . Cross-Table X-ray
Tx:	Mild = repair now Severe = colostomy, repair before toilet training
F/u:	**V**ertebra U/S Sacrum **A**nus X-ray **C**ardiac Echo **TE** Fistula X-ray with **E**sophageal Atresia coiled tube **R**enal VCUG **L**imb X-ray

MECONIUM ILEUS	
Path:	Cystic Fibrosis
Pt:	FTPM and . . . ~~+ prenatal screen~~ (didn't have a screen) ∅ prenatal care (undocumented)
Dx:	X-ray = dilated loops, gas filled plug Water soluble contrast (gastrografin enema)
Tx:	Water soluble contrast (gastrografin enema)
F/u:	Meconium peritonitis = perf ADEK vitamins Pancreatic enzymes Short stature

HIRSCHSPRUNG'S	
Path:	Failure of neuron migration = distal colon Absent inhibitor neurons = no relaxation
Pt:	Case 1 (90%): FTPM, explosive stool with DRE Case 2 (10%): Chronic constipation with overflow incontinence
Dx:	X-ray: Good bowel = dilated Bad bowel = normal If FTPM: Contrast Enema If Constipation: Anorectal manometry ↑ tone Best = Biopsy = absent neurons
Tx:	Surgery

VOLUNTARY CONSTIPATION	
Path:	Embarrassment or Pain Cognitive Impairment
Pt:	Toilet training OR school aged child Constipation with overflow incontinence Encopresis
Dx:	Clinical
Tx:	Bowel regimen (stool softener, motility) Disimpaction under anesthesia if necessary

Neonatal Jaundice

UNCONJUGATED	CONJUGATED
Lipid Soluble	Water Soluble
Can cross BBB	Cannot cross BBB
Kernicterus	NO kernicterus
NO urinary excretion	Urinary Excretion

PHYSIOLOGIC	PATHOLOGIC
Onset ≥ 72 hrs	Onset < 24 hrs
Bilirubin ↑ < 5/day (slow)	Bilirubin ↑ > 5/day (fast)
D. Bili < 10% Total	D. Bili > 10% Total
Resolves in 1 week (term) or 2 weeks (preterm)	Resolves in ≥ 1 week (term) or ≥ 2 weeks (preterm)

METABOLIC SYNDROMES	
Crigler–Najjar	NO UDP-glucuronyltransferase, Type I Die, Type II have unconjugated bili (very rare)
Gilbert's	↓ UDP-glucuronyltransferase, unconjugated bili (most common of these diseases)
Dubin-Johnson	Problem with excretion, conjugated hyperbilirubinemia; black liver
Rotor	Looks just like Dubin-Johnson, conjugated, No black liver, problem with storage

BREAST FEEDING	BREAST MILK JAUNDICE
< 7 days of life	> 10 days of life
Not enough feeding, slowing of gut, ↑ Bili Reabsorption	Enzyme inhibition by mother's milk; insufficient conjugation
↑ Feed Frequency	Phototherapy (if needed) and continuation of breast feeding OR supplement with formula x 1 week

pale stools (handwritten)

NEONATAL JAUNDICE	
Path:	Unconjugated causes kernicterus Conjugated implies structural lesion
Pt:	Baby will be yellow
Dx:	Transcutaneous sensor (screen) Bilirubin level (diagnostic)
Tx:	If Unconjugated: use BLUE LIGHT If Conjugated: evaluate for cause

obstructive (aka conjugated bili) more likely to be pathologic (handwritten)

Baby Emesis

TRACHEOESOPHAGEAL FISTULA

Path:	± Fistula ± Atresia Most common type C (blind pouch of esophagus with fistula from distal esophagus to trachea)
Pt:	Nonbiliary emesis day 0 Bubbling Gurgling
Dx:	NG Tube coils on X-ray
Tx:	Parenteral nutrition NG tube suction Surgery

PYLORIC STENOSIS

Path:	Hypertrophy of Pylorus Gastric Outlet Obstruction
Pt:	2-8 weeks, normal feeds → projectile Usually a boy * Olive-Shaped Mass * * Visible Peristaltic Waves *
Dx:	BMP = ↓ Cl, ↓ K, ↑ Bicarb U/S = Donut Sign
Tx:	FIX E-LYTES FIRST = IVF Pyloromyotomy

MALROTATION

Path:	Failure of rotation
Pt:	Normal uterine course No polyhydramnios No Down Syndrome
Dx:	X-ray = Double Bubble with NORMAL gas pattern beyond Upper GI Series
Tx:	NG tube decompression Surgery
F/u:	Volvulus; ischemia

DUODENAL ATRESIA

Path:	Failure to recannulate the duodenum
Pt:	+ Polyhydramnios + Down syndrome
Dx:	X-ray = Double Bubble AND no gas beyond
Tx:	Surgery

ANNULAR PANCREAS

Path:	Failure to recannulate the esophagus
Pt:	+ Polyhydramnios + Down syndrome
Dx:	X-ray = Double Bubble AND no gas beyond
Tx:	Surgery

INTESTINAL ATRESIA

Path:	Vascular compromise
Pt:	Mom = Cocaine use NO Down syndrome
Dx:	X-ray = double bubble with multiple air-fluid levels
Tx:	Surgery for baby Confront mom
F/u:	Short-gut

PEDS

Congenital Defects

CONGENITAL DIAPHRAGMATIC HERNIA	
Path:	Bowel in chest Hypoplastic Lungs
Pt:	Scaphoid Abdomen Pulmonary Distress day 0 Bowel sounds in chest
Dx:	X-ray (babygram)
Tx:	Cardiopulmonary stabilization Pulmonary Surfactant Surgical Repair

GASTROSCHISIS	
Path:	Extrusion of bowel NO membrane
Pt:	RIGHT of midline NO membrane (loose bowel)
Dx:	Clinical
Tx:	Silo
F/u:	Fluid shifts big problem

OMPHALOCELE	
Path:	Extrusion of bowel Intact membrane
Pt:	MIDLINE YES membrane (contained sack)
Dx:	Clinical
Tx:	Silo
F/u:	Fluid shifts but not as fast

EXSTROPHY OF THE BLADDER	
Path:	Bladder through the skin
Pt:	MIDLINE defect Wet with urine Red or shining No bowel seen
Dx:	Clinical
Tx:	Surgically

BILIARY ATRESIA	
Path:	Failure of the biliary tree to recanalize
Pt:	Persistent or worsening jaundice at 2 weeks Direct Hyperbili
Dx:	Ultrasound = absence of ducts HIDA scan after phenobarb = no contrast in GI
Tx:	Surgical (hepatoportoenterostomy)
F/u:	Fatal if not corrected

liver biopsy

NEURAL TUBE DEFECTS	
Path:	Genetic Syndromes FOLATE deficiency Failure of the caudal neural tube to fuse
Pt:	Occulta: Tuft of hair only Meningocele: extrusion of meninges without cord Myelomeningocele: extrusion of meninges with cord
Dx:	Prenatal + AFP screen + Ultrasound in utero No Prenatal Care + Visual inspection
Tx:	Surgery
F/u:	Chiari Type II with Myelomeningocele Hydrocephalus can lead to learning disabilities

non comm

CLEFT LIP / CLEFT PALATE	
Path:	Failure of growth and fusion of the underlying structures
Pt:	Spectrum: lip through uvula Spectrum: superficial through transmural Spectrum: unilateral, bilateral, midline
Dx:	Clinical
Tx:	Surgically
F/u:	Cosmetic deformity Failure to thrive from inability to latch (feed)

Can be part of Patau

Well Child Visit

	Gross Motor	Fine Motor	Speech	Social
DEVELOPMENTAL MILESTONES				
2mo	**Lift Head**	Tracks past mid	coos	**Social Smile**
4mo	**Roll Over**	Clumsy Grasp	Laughs, Squeals	Looks around
6mo	**Sit up**	Rakes	Babbles	**Stranger Anxiety**
1yr	**Walk**	Pincer Grasp	**1-word**	**Separation Anxiety**
2yr	**Steps**		**2-word**	**2-step commands**
3yr	**Trike**	**Circle**	**3-word**	-------
4yr	**Hop**	**Cross**	**4-word**	--------
5yr	**Skip**	**Triangle**	**5-word**	--------

VACCINES	
MMRV	Pneumococcal
Hep A / B	Meningococcal
DTaP	HPV
HiB	Flu

FAILURE TO THRIVE	
Head Circumference	Last to go
Height	Lost between
Weight	First to go
Organic	*Non-Organic*
Genetic (CF)	Formula
Cardiac Disease	Feeding
Pyloric Stenosis	Frequency
GERD	

RED FLAGS OF ABUSE	
Injury	*Child*
Suspicious Shape	Injured Infant
Suspicious Location	Comfort from nurses
Severity	Comfort from staff

SAFETY	
Prevent Trauma	*SIDS*
Car Seats	Sleep on Back
Booster Seats	Don't share beds
Seatbelts	Smoking Cessation
NO Trampolines	
Eliminate Guns	
Fence pools	

PEDS

Vaccinations

CONTRAINDICATIONS	
Egg Allergy	Nothing made with eggs except: - Influenza* - Yellow fever
Immuno↓ or Pregnant	No live vaccines: - MMRV - Live attenuated influenza (IN)
Anaphylaxis	Never get that vaccine again
OK to give vaccine again if . . .	Prior local reactions, current illness or fever, family history of ___, autism fear

* US Intramuscular Flu no longer made with eggs
* Intranasal live attenuated available just in case

VACCINES	
Hep B	Mom:⊕Baby: **Hep B Ig** and **Hep B Vacc NOW** Mom: ⊖Baby: Hep B within 2 months Mom: ? Baby: Hep B NOW, check mom's HBsAg
DTaP	Kids get 5 doses: **3 doses in 1st year** and **2 doses** between 1-4 years Td (booster) or Tdap at least once in Adolescence and every **q10yrs** Need **3 total doses** lifetime (see below)
Hib	Disease **does not** confer immunity in those < 2y so give Hib vaccine. Does not cover non-typeable. Hib causes epiglottitis + meningitis
MMRV	Vaccine and booster before school
Pneumo coccal	Two types: 23 and 13 valent Complete 13 as infant, add 23 if + risk factors to all **immunocompromised** and **asplenic** pts
Meningo coccal	To **everyone** vs. meningitis . . . Required for **College** and **Military**
HPV	All boys and girls age 9-26 years Prevents cancer
Hep A/B	2 doses for A 3 doses for B Pick up where you left off
Flu	Everyone. Period Health care workers before winter months Given annually

MANAGING A WOUND WITH < 3 LIFETIME DOSES (OR UNKNOWN)	
Type of Wound	
Clean	*Dirty*
Tdap	Tdap +TIG
TIMING DOESN'T MATTER IF < 3 Lifetime Doses	

MANAGING A WOUND WITH ≥ 3 LIFETIME DOSES	
Type of Wound	
Clean	*Dirty*
≥ 10y Tdap	≥ 5y Tdap
< 10y Home	< 5y Home
No TIG needed if ≥ 3 lifetime doses	

DISEASES	
Pertussis	Catarrhal stage (inconspicuous) Paroxysmal Phase (coughing spells, whoops) Resolution Phase (regular cold symptoms)
Diphtheria	Grey pseudomembrane in oropharynx Airway, Antibiotics, Antitoxin
Tetanus	Dirty Wound, Lock Jaw, Spasms TIG (Block toxin) and Toxoid (Vaccinate) Lethal dose < Immune Dose Tube, Sedate, MTZ
Varicella	**No pox parties** → vaccinate instead Kids get MMRV = no chickenpox Adults, no "V" = Shingles = Varicella @ 60
HPV	**Boys** and **Girls** aged **9-26** Does **prevent cancer** Does **NOT** ↑ sex, STI, pregnancy, etc.
Rotavirus	Oral Contraindicated in intussusception
Measles Mumps Rubella	See viral exanthems

Preventable Trauma

BURNS
1st Degree = epidermis only, ⊕ **pain** ⊕ **erythema** 2nd Degree = epi + dermis, ⊕ **pain** ⊕ **blisters** ⊕ **erythema** 3rd Degree = through dermis, **white and painless** with surrounding 2nd degree burns

Parkland Formula	%BSA x Kg x 4 2° and 3° only	50% in 8 hrs 50% in 16 hrs

Rule of 9s

Head	9 + 9 = 18	
Front Thorax	9 + 9 = 18	
Back Thorax	9 + 9 = 18	
Arms	L = 9 + R = 9 = 18	
Legs	9 + 9 + 9 = 27	
Genitals	1	

Front   Back

HEAD TRAUMA			
Disease	*Trauma*	*Symptoms*	*CT*
Epidural Hematoma	Temple Trauma	⊕LOC with Lucid Interval	Biconvex "lens"
Subdural Hematoma	Major trauma or abuse	⊕LOC Ø Lucidity	Concave "crescent"
Cerebral Contusion	Major Trauma	⊕LOC	Punctate Hemorrhage

DROWNING PREVENTION	
Limit Access	**Locked Gates** Surrounding all pools
Supervision	Supervision near **tubs**, pools, and **tanks**
Flotation	Use **life jackets**, NOT arm floaties
Up Risk	**Too young to know** **Too drunk to remember** **(adolescents)**

HEAD TRAUMA PREVENTION	
Helmets	Helmets **in sports and on bikes**
Car Safety	**Rear-facing** car seats **day 0-2 years** **Booster seat** until 4'9" and 8-12 years old **Seat belts** in cars for everyone in every seat
Trampolines	**Eliminate** trampolines - Nets, soft ground, water, etc. DON'T COUNT

GUN AND CHEMICAL SAFETY	
Best	**Eliminate** them from the home
OK	Keep them out of reach—**store up high** Keep them **locked** in a **safe** or locked cabinet do NOT depend on "child-proof" lids
Guns	**Ammo** stored separately from **Weapon** Store guns **unloaded**

SEVERITY OF CONCUSSION TO TREATMENT		
Mild		*Severe*
None	FND	Positive
< 60 seconds	LOC	> 60 seconds
None, Improving	Headache	Present or worsening
None	Amnesia	Retrograde or Anterograde
No CT		CT scan
Discharge Home		Observe in house
Treatment regardless of severity		
Step-Wise Return to play Sleep → go to school → homework → practice → play		

PEDS

Abuse

ABUSE	VS.	NEGLECT
+ Sxs		- Sxs
Intentional		Absence
Active		Passive

RISK FACTORS FOR ABUSE	
Child	Parental
Intellectual Disability	Those who were abused
Premature Birth	Single Parent
Physical Disability	Young Parent
Cognitive Disability	Low SES

HOW TO SPOT ABUSE	
Consideration	Things to look for
Fractures:	Skull or Clavicle Femur, especially spiral Rib fractures in infants Different stages of healing
Bruises:	Different Stages of healing
Burns:	Feet, ankles (Dunk) Buttocks only (Dunk) Punctate circular burns (cigarettes)
Sexual:	Any STD in any child ever Vaginal or Anal trauma
Behavior:	Not crying in the presence of parent Running from care-giver Receiving comfort from health-care provider rather than care-giver

WHAT TO DO IF YOU SUSPECT ABUSE	
Element	Considerations
Certainty:	Certainty is NOT required
The Family:	Tell the family why you are doing it and that you are required by law to do so
The Child:	Hospitalize child if no safe alternative exists
The Abuser:	Separate abuser from child if obvious Separate parent-child unit from a common abuser
Behavior:	Offer resources and support that allows families and care givers to understand disease process, provide emotional, economic, and physical support
CPS	Must Report

ALTE / BRUE and SIDS

ALTE Definition
Frightened observer plus any combination of: - Change in color: red, blue, or pale - Change in muscle tone: hypertonic or hypotonic - Change in respirations: choking, gagging, or apnea

FEATURES BY ETIOLOGY	
Seizures	Eye deviation, limb-jerking
Infection	Temperature instability Fussy baby
Cardiac	Difficulty with feeding Murmur Failure to thrive
Abuse	Evidence of trauma Femur, Skull fracture

BRUE Definition
< 1 year old + < 1 min duration + . . . - Change in color: red, blue, or pale - Change in muscle tone: hypertonic or hypotonic - Change in respirations: choking, gagging, or apnea - Change in responsiveness

STRATIFYING BRUE	
Low-Risk	High-Risk
No History	History suggestive of dz
No Physical	Physical suggestive of dz
No CPR	CPR performed
1st Time, non-recurring	Multiple, Recurring
Age, Term > 60 days	Not old enough
Age, > 32 wk GA Preterm And ≥ 45 wk PC	
Action	Action
Reassurance only	NO SET WORKUP Go after workup based on history and physical

SIDS Prevention	
Back to sleep	Flatten occiput
Don't share a bed	
Smoking cessation	

Infectious Rashes

ERYTHEMA INFECTIOSUM	
Path:	Parvovirus 19
Pt:	Slapped-Cheek Rash
Dx:	Clinical
Tx:	None
F/u:	Aplastic Crisis in sickle cell Hydrops Fetalis if in utero

MEASLES	
Path:	Measles virus (a paramyxovirus)

Pt:	Cough, Coryza, Conjunctivitis,
	    Koplik Spots
	Fever AND Rash
	    - Starts on face spreads to
	        extremities

Tx:	Supportive (PPx Vaccinate)
F/u:	Subacute Sclerosing Panencephalitis

RUBELLA	
Path:	Rubella
Pt:	Fever BEFORE Rash Starts on face, spread to toes Prodrome of Lymphadenitis
Tx:	Supportive (PPx Vaccinate)
F/u:	Congenital: Heart, Deafness, Cataracts

ROSEOLA	
Path:	HHV-6
Pt:	Fever BEFORE Rash (> 104) Starts on trunk, spreads outwards
F/u:	Febrile seizures

VARICELLA = CHICKEN POX	
Path:	Varicella Zoster
Pt:	Wide spread Vesicles on an erythematous base Different stages of healing

Tx:	Supportive, antivirals for teens
	    and those with lung issues (PPx
	    Vaccinate)

F/u:	Shingles

VARICELLA = SHINGLES	
Path:	Reactivated Varicella, non-vaccinated adults
Pt:	Pain precedes rash Vesicles on an erythematous base Does NOT cross midline Confined to a dermatome
Tx:	Antiviral if immunocompromised (PPx Vaccinate)
F/u:	Post-herpetic neuralgia

MUMPS	
Path:	Mumps virus
Pt:	Bilateral Swelling Orchitis in pubertal males
Dx:	Clinical
Tx:	Vaccinate
F/u:	Infertility

HAND-FOOT-MOUTH	
Path:	Coxsackie A
Pt:	Nonspecific Prodrome Vesicle on erythematous base but only on the hands, feet, and mouth
Dx:	Clinical

MOLLUSCUM CONTAGIOSUM	
Path:	Poxvirus
Pt:	Flesh-colored Central umbilication Trunk, Arms, Diaper
Dx:	Clinical
Tx:	Supportive

SCARLET FEVER	
Path:	Group Strep A
Pt:	Fever, Sore throat Desquamating sandpaper rash Trunk and spreads outwards
Dx:	Streptolysin O

Tx:	Penicillin prevents rheumatic
	    fever but not post-strep
	    glomerulonephritis

Acute Allergic Reactions

ANAPHYLAXIS	
Path:	IgE Mediated Life Threatening
Pt:	Rash (urticarial) AND Airway Edema HYPOTENSION
Dx:	Clinical

Tx:	Epi 1:1000 IM "epi pen" …
	    Then H1/H2 blockers
	    Then Steroids

F/u:	Avoid Triggers

URTICARIA	
Path:	IgE Mediated Rash only

Pt:	Rash (urticarial)
	    - Erythema
	    - Wheal
	NO Hypotension

Dx:	Clinical
Tx:	Topical or oral antihistamines Avoidance of trigger If anaphylaxis, treat that

ANGIOEDEMA	
Path:	Non IgE Mediated Swelling Medication Induced C1 Esterase Deficiency

Pt:	Swelling can involve mouth, throat,
	    tongue which makes it life
	    threatening

Dx:	Clinical
Tx:	Airway protection Stop the offending agent (ACE- inhibitor)
F/u:	C1 Esterase Deficiency gets FFP H1/H2 blockers and steroids probably don't help

Chronic Allergic Reactions

ALLERGIC RHINITIS	
Path:	Seasonal (dander / pollen exposure) Perennial (pets, dust, indoor mold)
Pt:	Allergic Shiners (dark eyes) Allergic Salute (nasal crease) Pale, Boggy Mucosa Polyps Cobblestoning

Dx:	Identify and remove triggers
	    - Pets
	    - Carpets
	    - Parents Smoking
	Skin testing if severe or refractory
	    to trigger

Tx:	Avoid Triggers
	Antihistamines
	    - Mild-Moderate = 2nd gen
	        (Loratadine, Fexofenadine,
	        Cetirizine)
	    - Moderate-Severe = Intranasal
	        Corticosteroids

ALLERGIC CONJUNCTIVITIS	
Path:	Same as Rhinitis

Pt:	Same as rhinitis, except it's the eyes
	    Injection
	    Chemosis
	    Shiners

Dx:	Clinical

Tx:	Avoid triggers
	Mast Cell Stabilizers and
	    antihistamines instead of intranasal
	    steroids

FOOD ALLERGENS	

Path:	Triggers:
	    Outgrows: Wheat, Soy, milk, eggs
	    For Life: nuts, shellfish, seafood

Pt:	Atopic Dermatitis N/V/D Anaphylaxis possible (nuts, shellfish)
Dx:	Food trial
Tx:	Epi Pen for Anaphylaxis Avoidance of trigger

MILK PROTEIN ALLERGY	
Path:	Soy / Formula
Pt:	N/V/D Bloody Bowel Movements Failure to Thrive
Dx:	Clinical
Tx:	Cow's Milk Formula or Breastfeed

ENT

ACUTE OTITIS MEDIA	
Path:	URI Bugs = Strep, Moraxella, H. flu Middle Ear
Pt:	Unilateral ear pain Relief of pain on pulling pinna Loss of Light reflex Erythema, Tympanic Effusion
Dx:	Pneumatic Insufflation
Tx:	1st: Amoxicillin Recur: Amoxicillin-Clavulanate Re-Recur: Tympanoplasty PCN all: Cefdinir → Azithromycin
F/u:	Mastoiditis

ACUTE OTITIS EXTERNA	
Path:	Outer Ear Swimmer's = Pseudomonas Digital = *Staph. aureus*
Pt:	Unilateral ear pain NO relief of pain on pulling pinna Angry Erythematous Canal
Dx:	Clinical
Tx:	Spontaneously resolves
F/u:	Toxic, malignant otitis externa, use Cipro and steroid ear drops

MASTOIDITIS	
Path:	Complication of Ear Infections
Pt:	Acute Otitis Media AND Posterior bulging of mastoid Anteriorly rotated ear
Dx:	Clinical . . . CT scan (not needed)
Tx:	Surgical drainage

BACTERIAL SINUSITIS	
Path:	URI bugs (same as OM)
Pt:	Congestion Bilateral Purulent Rhinorrhea Facial Tap = Pain
Dx:	Clinical ~~XR = Air-Fluid levels~~ ~~CT = opacification~~
Tx:	Supportive EXCEPT - Temp ≥ 38° C - Worsening - Duration > 10 days Amoxicillin + Clavulanate
F/u:	CT scan for recurrence Foreign Body for young kids

COMMON COLD	
Path:	Rhinovirus, transmitted by large droplets
Pt:	Congestion, Non-toxic < 10 days, No purulence
Dx:	Clinical ~~XR,~~ PCR/IF on washings ~~CT,~~ ~~bacterial culture~~
Tx:	Supportive

PHARYNGITIS		
Path:	Viral (most common) Group Strep A (Rheumatic Fever)	
Pt:	Sore Throat, Odynophagia	
	Cough (absent)	+1
	Exudates	+1
	Nodes (adenopathy)	+1
	Temp ≥ 38° C	+1
	OR age < 14 +1 OR age > 44	-1
Dx:	≤ 1: Supportive 2-3: Rapid strep (culture or treat) ≥ 4: Treat as strep	
Tx:	Amoxicillin or Penicillin	

FOREIGN BODIES	
Path:	Kids stick things places
Pt:	Unilateral Purulent discharge Unilateral Otitis Externa Aspiration
Dx:	Clinical, CXR
Tx:	Retrieval
F/u:	If insect gets in: - Lidocaine and retrieval - ~~Light in ear~~ (NEVER DO THIS)

EPISTAXIS	
Path:	Digital trauma (nose picking)
Pt:	Unilateral bleeding, < 30 minutes
Dx:	Clinical
Tx:	Ice pack, lean forward Cauterize anterior bleeds Pack posterior bleeds

CHOANAL ATRESIA	
Path:	Atresia or Stenosis of passage from nose to throat
Pt:	Blue while feeding, pink while crying Childhood snore
Dx:	Catheter fails to pass through the nose
Tx:	Scope and Surgery

Upper Airway

CROUP	
Path:	Parainfluenza
Pt:	3 mo – 3 yrs old Viral prodrome precedes Seal-Like barking cough interspersed with stridor
Dx:	Clinical X-ray = Steeple Sign
Tx:	Mild: misting Moderate: Racemic Epi, Steroids, O_2 Severe: Admit for Oxygen support

RETROPHARYNGEAL ABSCESS	
Path:	Oral flora URI bugs
Pt:	SICK Rapid onset high spiking fevers Drooling, neck extended Hot-Potato-Voice ("muffled") * Unilateral anterior chain nodes * * Tender palpable mass *
Dx:	CT Scan max/face/neck
Tx:	Incision and drainage, IV Abx

BACTERIAL TRACHEITIS	
Path:	Strep and Staph
Pt:	5-7 yrs old Croup that doesn't get any better with Croup treatment; also more insidious
Dx:	Clinical X-ray = Steeple Sign Tracheal Culture
Tx:	IV Abx
F/u:	ENT to bronch/scope/get tracheal culture

PERITONSILLAR ABSCESS	
Path	Oral Flora URI bugs
Pt	> 10 years old Hot-Potato-Voice ("muffled") Drooling, Sore throat * Uvular Deviation *
Dx:	Clinical
Tx:	Incision and drainage, IV Abx

EPIGLOTTITIS	
Path:	Hib (Hib vaccine has dropped incidence)
Pt:	6-12 years, unvaccinated SICK Rapid onset high spiking fevers Drooling, Tripoding Accessory muscles Hot-Potato-Voice ("muffled")
Dx:	Clinical Direct visualization of cherry-red epiglottis during airway X-ray = Thumbprint
Tx:	Secure airway in the OR. DO NOT TOUCH THE EPIGLOTTIS IV Abx after airway secured = Cefuroxime, Ceftriaxone

Lower Airway

FOREIGN BODY ASPIRATION	
Path:	Kids put things places
Pt:	Sudden onset dyspnea Unsupervised child Stridor = Extrathoracic Wheeze = Intrathoracic

Dx:	1st: CXR PA and Lateral
	  - Coin sign AP rules out trachea
	  - Coin sign lateral nonspecific
	Best: Rigid Bronchoscope

Tx:	Retrieval

F/u:	High Risk:
	  - Kids < 3 years old
	  - Foods: peanuts, M&Ms, hot dogs

ASTHMA	
Path:	Reversible obstructive lung disease
Pt:	Wheezing, dyspnea during attacks Normal between attacks Asthma, Allergy, and Atopy

Dx:	PFTs
	  - ↓ FEV1/FVC
	  - reversible with bronchodilators
	  - inducible with methacholine

Tx:	Chronic Escalation
	  - SABA
	  - SABA + ICS
	  - SABA + ↑ ICS
	  - SABA + ↑ ICS + LABA
	  … add steroids
	  … LTA are oral adjuncts
	Acute Exacerbation
	  - Peak flow before and after
	  - Albuterol / Ipratropium
	  - IV steroids
	  - Maybe magnesium
	  - Maybe subQ epi

F/u:	Remove allergens
	  - Pets
	  - Carpets
	  - Smoking (parents)

PNEUMONIA	
Path:	Typical, Atypical, Viral
Pt:	Pre-school = Viral School or older = Bacterial Fever, Cough, Consolidation on CXR
Dx:	CXR
Tx:	Amoxicillin or Azithromycin
F/u:	Internal Medicine—Infectious ID

BRONCHIOLITIS	
Path:	Inflammatory disorder of small airways Viral Infxn = RSV
Pt:	Very young < 2 years old Trouble feeding

Dx:	~~CXR~~ (normal)
	Rapid Antigen testing from a
	  Nasopharyngeal swab (yes, but
	  don't)

Tx:	Supportive—IV fluids/NG feeds,
	  oxygen
	NO:
	  - Steroids
	  - β-agonists
	  - Antibiotics

F/u:	RSV Bronchiolitis is all supportive
	  care. Nothing works; just get the
	  kids through it.

CYSTIC FIBROSIS	
Path:	CFTR or CCTR mutation, Autosomal Recessive

Pt:	Prenatal Screen positive
	  - most diagnosis
	No prenatal screen (immigrant)
	  - Failure to thrive
	  - Meconium ileus
	  - Frequent Respiratory infections
	  - Baby has salty skin

Dx:	Sweat Chloride Test
	  - > 40 neonates
	  - > 60 in others

Tx:	Pulmonary Toilet Pneumonia = Pseudomonas Vit ADEK Pancreatic Enzymes
F/u:	Short stature Limited life expectancy

GI Bleed

NECROTIZING ENTEROCOLITIS	
Path:	Dying gut
Pt:	Premature neonate in ICU Bloody bowel movement
Dx:	X-ray = Pneumatosis Intestinalis
Tx:	NPO, IVF, TPN IV Abx
F/u:	Other diseases of prematurity

ANAL FISSURE	
Path:	Tear in anal mucosa
Pt:	Visual inspection Iatrogenic in the neonate, well baby
Dx:	Clinical

Tx:	Reassurance
	(babies are incontinent of stool,
	   the stool is soft, and it will heal
	   spontaneously)

INTUSSUSCEPTION	
Path:	Telescoping of bowel Vascular compromise
Pt:	Abrupt onset Colicky pain Knee-chest position = relief * Sausage-Shaped mass in RUQ * * Currant Jelly Stool * (too late)
Dx:	X-ray = Perforation, obstruction U/S = Target sign (aka Donut) Air-Enema best test

Tx:	Air-Enema usually curative
	Surgery if
	   - Peritoneal
	   - Perforation
	   - Failed Air-Enema

F/u:	90% of kids have no lead point 90% of adults have a mass lead point

MECKEL'S DIVERTICULUM	
Path:	Remnant of the Vitelline Duct = gastric mucosa (omphalomesenteric duct)

Pt:	"Colon Cancer" at 2 years old
	   - Painless, Intermittent
	      Hematochezia
	   - Iron deficiency anemia
	   - FOBT +
	Rule of 2s
	   - < 2 years old at diagnosis
	   - < 2 % of population
	   - 2x boys: girls
	   - 2 feet from ileocecal valve
	   - 2 inches in length

Dx:	Meckel's Scan = Technetium-99
Tx:	Surgery
F/u:	Teenagers get diagnosed with CT scans

DISTRACTORS → REASSURANCE ONLY	
Swallowed maternal blood	Apt test, Melena after delivery
Swallowed self-blood	Epistaxis history
Dietary	Iron, beets, medications

OTHER NOTABLES	
Crohn's	Watery diarrhea, weight loss, fistulas EGD + Colon = Skip Lesions Medications to control Surgery only for fistulas
UC	Bloody diarrhea Colon = continuous lesions Hemicolectomy curative @ 8y, q1y colonoscopy until resected

Infectious
Colitis
	Fever and blood bowel
	   movement
	Lactoferrin, WBC, Stool
	   culture

Milk-Protein Allergy	Change to Hydrolyzed formula

CT Surgery

LEFT TO RIGHT SHUNTS
↑ Pulmonary Flow
↑ Pulmonary Vasculature on X-ray
↑ Pulmonary Pressures
Right Ventricular Hypertrophy
Eisenmenger's (reversal to Right to Left)
"D" Diseases: ASD, VSD, PDA

RIGHT TO LEFT SHUNTS
↓ Pulmonary Flow
↓ Pulmonary Vasculature on X-ray
Deoxygenated Blood in periphery
Blue Baby Syndrome
Fatal if not corrected
The "T" Diseases: Tetralogy, TGA, TA, TAPVR

ATRIAL SEPTAL DEFECT	
Path:	Ostium Primum (rare) Ostium Secundum (more common)
Pt:	Fixed Split S2 Most Common Murmur > 1 year old
Dx:	Echo
Tx:	Surgical closure

VENTRICULAR SEPTAL DEFECT	
Path:	Hole between the two ventricles
Pt:	Harsh Holosystolic Murmur in a neonate . . . but the worst defects have no murmur Most common congenital heart disease . . . likely get fixed or die before 1 year Failure to thrive, Down syndrome
Dx:	Echo
Tx:	If CHF, Failure to thrive, dyspnea = fix now If none of those things = fix only if increased pulmonary blood flow
F/u:	Surgical closure likely required, may spontaneously resolve

PATENT DUCTUS ARTERIOSUS	
Path:	Ductus arteriosus remains open, a connection between aorta and pulmonary artery
Pt:	Continuous Machinery-Like Murmur
Dx:	Echo
Tx:	If no CHF → Indomethacin = Ends the PDA (preterm infants only) If yes CHF → Surgical Closure If cyanotic defect → prostaglandins to sustain PDA
F/u:	Close as necessary, but many that persist are clinically insignificant

Truncus Arteriosus, Tricuspid Atresia, and Total Anomalous Pulmonary Venous Return are intentionally NOT included in this section because they are too low yield for Step 2.

TETRALOGY OF FALLOT	
Path:	1: Overriding Aorta 2: Pulmonary Stenosis 3: Right ventricular Hypertrophy 4:Ventricular Septal Defect "Endocardial Cushion defect"
Pt:	Most common cyanotic disease of children because TGA babies die or get fixed "Tet Spells" cyanosis relieved by squatting
Dx:	1st: Boot Shaped heart on X-ray Best: Echocardiogram
Tx:	Surgical Correction
F/u:	Associated with Down's Syndrome

TRANSPOSITION OF THE GREAT ARTERIES	
Path:	Heart fails to twist Pulmonary Artery and Vein both connected to the left heart and lungs Aorta and Vena Cava both connected to the right heart and periphery TWO separate circulatory systems connected only by ductus arteriosus
Pt:	Blue baby day 1—you will not miss this Mom is a diabetic at the start of pregnancy ~~Gestational Diabetes~~ (not a risk factor)
Dx:	Echo
Tx:	Prostaglandins to support PDA Surgical Correction

COARCTATION OF AORTA	
Path:	Turner Syndrome
Pt:	Hypertension in upper extremities, hypotension in lower extremities in a child Claudication (crying with crawling or walking)
Dx:	Clinical: Blood Pressures in all extremities X-ray shows rib notching (not diagnostic) Aortogram
Tx:	Surgical Correction

PEDS

Orthopedics

DEVELOPMENTAL DYSPLASIA OF THE HIP	
Age:	Newborn
Pt:	Clicky hip during the neonatal evaluation, the Ortolani and Barlow maneuvers
Dx:	Ultrasound @ 4-6 weeks
Tx:	Harness

LEGG-CALVE-PERTHES	
Age:	6
Pt:	Insidious onset antalgic gait
Dx:	X-ray
Tx:	Cast

SLIPPED-CAPITAL FEMORAL EPIPHYSIS	
Age:	13
Pt:	Fat kid going through a growth spurt. Non-traumatic knee pain
Dx:	Frog-Leg X-ray
Tx:	Surgery (urgently)

SEPTIC HIP	
Age:	ANY AGE
Pt:	Fever and Joint Pain, especially after another febrile illness or unprotected sex
Dx:	Arthrocentesis (> 50,000 WBC)
Tx:	Drainage and Abx

TRANSIENT SYNOVITIS	
Age:	ANY AGE
Pt:	4-6 weeks after a viral illness Joint pain WITHOUT fever, leukocytosis, inflammatory makers
Dx:	History
Tx:	Supportive

OSGOOD-SCHLATTER'S DISEASE	
Path:	Osteochondrosis
Pt:	Teenage athlete with knee pain, swelling and eventually palpable nodule on the tibia
Dx:	Clinical
Tx:	Rest + Cast (aka stop exercising, curative) Work through it (palpable nodule)

SCOLIOSIS	
Path:	Spinal deformity (left to right) - not Lordosis, not kyphosis
Pt:	Teenage girl who can present with either moderate: cosmetic severe: shortness of breath
Dx:	Adam's Test is positive (have the girl lean forward and see asymmetry)
Tx:	No therapy Brace Surgery with rods

OSTEOGENIC SARCOMA	
Path:	Retinoblastoma gene, associated with retinoblastoma of the eye
Pt:	Bone pain in a pre-teen / teenager Retinoblastoma at birth (neonatal)
Dx:	1st: X-ray = distal femur, sunburst pattern Then: MRI Best: Biopsy
Tx:	Surgery

FRACTURE IN KIDS	
Path:	Fractures can occur for any reason, trauma, fall, and child abuse. You must think of the growth plate, a consideration not in adults
Pt:	Leg pain, trauma
Dx:	X-ray
Tx:	Involves growth plate → ORIF Does not involve growth plate → Cast

Orthopedics

EWING'S SARCOMA	
Path:	Translocation t(11:22)
Pt:	Bone pain in a pre-teen/teenager No risk factor
Dx:	1st: X-ray = midshaft, onion-skin pattern Then: MRI Best: Biopsy
Tx:	Surgery

SPECIAL CONSIDERATIONS FOR PEDI FRACTURES	
External Fixation	Closed, simple, aligned, **No growth plate**
Open reduction and internal fixation	Comminuted Angular Displaced Open **Or involves the growth plate**

Peds Psych

*For Pediatric Psych, see Peds Behavioral
and Neurodevelopment in Psychiatry.*

Sickle Cell

SICKLE CELL DISEASE	
Path:	HgbSS—Autosomal recessive Valine for Glutamic acid on 6th Position
Pt:	Asplenism Vasoocclusive Crisis Chronic Pain Chronic Anemia Pigmented Gallstones
Dx:	Sickle Cells on Smear Hgb Electrophoresis
Tx:	Hydroxyurea (↑ HgbF) Iron, Folate Penicillin until age 5

F/u:	Hemosiderosis from transfusions =
	     deferoxamine / deferasirox
	Asplenism = Pneumovax
	Avascular Necrosis of the hip =
	     Conservative attempted → surgery

VASOOCCLUSIVE CRISIS	
Path:	Sickling cells = ischemia and hemolysis
Pt:	Acute Pain Elevated Bilirubin, Elevated Reticulocytes Jaundice
Dx:	Blood Smear = Sickled Cells
Tx:	IVF, Pain Control

INDICATIONS FOR EXCHANGE TRANSFUSION
Priapism
Focal Neurologic Deficit, Stroke
Acute Chest (Chest Pain, Pulm Edema)

SICKLE VARIANTS	
HgbS-β^0	The worst
HgbSS	Sickle cell disease
HgbS-β^+	Milder
HgbSC	Almost not a disease
HgbS trait	Not a disease (carrier)

CONSIDERATION OF COMPLICATIONS	
Asplenism	PCN until 5 Vaccine for Strep
Iron overload	Deferoxamine
Avascular Necrosis	Conservative then surgery
Sickled HgbSS	Hydroxyurea
Anemia	Folate
Pain	Analgesics (opiates)
Osteomyelitis	Staph first, then Salmonella

PEDS

Ophthalmology

Type	Time	Purulent	Problems	Tx
Chemical	24 hrs	Non-purulent	Bilateral	Observation (caused by silver nitrate PPx)
Gonorrhea	Day 2-5	Purulent	Bilateral, Check for systemic illness!	Ceftriaxone IM
Chlamydia	Day 5-14	Muco-purulent	Unilateral then Bilateral	Erythromycin PO
			Associated with pneumonia	No topical antibiotics

RETINOBLASTOMA	
Path:	Rb gene mutation
Pt:	Newborn screen in the neonatal unit with an abnormal light reflex
Dx:	Red reflex (normal) = Pure White Retina "white thing in the BACK of the eye"
Tx:	Surgery ~~Radiation Therapy~~ (NEVER)
F/u:	Osteosarcoma

AMBLYOPIA	
Path:	Cortical Blindness
Pt:	Strabismus, Cataracts, another cause, leads to cortical blindness
Dx:	None
Tx:	None Fix the problem that could lead to cortical blindness

STRABISMUS	
Path:	"Lazy eye"
Pt:	Baby with one eye that focuses while the other does not Almost ALWAYS a photograph question
Dx:	Light reflects at different points on both eyes
Tx:	If present at birth - Patch the good eye - Surgery if all else fails Glasses if developed after birth

CONGENITAL CATARACTS	
Path:	Present at birth → TORCH infections Not present at birth → Galactosemia
Pt:	White cloudy lesions in front of their eye "white thing in FRONT of the eye"
Dx:	Clinical
Tx:	Surgical Removal

RETINOPATHY OF PREMATURITY	
Path:	Premature baby, oxygen toxicity
Pt:	Suspect in any premature neonate especially if any of the "other 3" are present
Dx:	Ophtho Exam = growths on retina
Tx:	Laser Ablation
F/u:	The "other three" Necrotizing Enterocolitis Bronchopulmonary Dysplasia Intraventricular Hemorrhage

This is a duplicate from surgery.

Urology

POSTERIOR URETHRAL VALVES	
Path:	Difficulty getting urine out Redundant tissue
Pt:	No urinary output + distended bladder, day 0 of life ± Oligohydramnios (prenatal U/S) ± ↑ Cr (mom clears)
Dx:	U/S = Hydro Catheter = large volume diuresis VCUG = negative reflux
Tx:	Catheter = relieve obstruction Surgery = resolve problem

HYPOSPADIAS / EPISPADIAS	
Path:	The scrotum "zips up" lopsided Hypo = under = Ventral urethra Epi = top = Dorsal urethra
Pt:	Cosmetic deformity Epi can lead to incontinence
Dx:	Clinical
Tx:	NEVER CIRCUMCISE, rebuild using foreskin

URETEROPELVIC JUNCTION OBSTRUCTION	
Path:	Narrow lumen "obstruction" to high flow
Pt:	Teenager on first alcohol binge gets colicky abdominal pain that spontaneously resolves
Dx:	U/S: hydronephrosis without hydroureter VCUG = no reflux
Tx:	Surgery ± stenting
F/u:	Ureterovesicular junction obstruction would have hydro of the entire side

ECTOPIC URETER (FORMERLY LOW IMPLANTATION)	
Path:	One good ureter = normal function One janky ureter = constant leak
Pt:	Boys: asymptomatic Girls: "normal" bladder function AND constant leak
Dx:	U/S: No hydro VCUG = no reflux Radionucleotide scan for renal function
Tx:	Reimplant

VESICOURETERAL REFLUX	
Path:	Retrograde flow to ureters Bacteria ascend
Pt:	Prenatal U/S = Hydro Recurrent UTI / Pyelo at young age
Dx:	U/S = Hydro VCUG = reflux
Tx:	Low grade = abx Ultimately = surgery

URO TEST	WHY
U/S	Hydro or no hydro
VCUG	Reflux or no reflux
CT Scan	Extraluminal lesions (IV contrast) Trauma (IV contrast) Nephrolithiasis (no contrast)
Cystoscopy	Intraluminal lesions Stent intervention
IVP	Never the right answer

HEMATURIA	
Microscopic	Likely self-limiting, investigate if persists.
Dysmorphic RBC, RBC Casts	Glomerulonephritis, lean on the U/A and maybe a biopsy (nephritic syndrome)
Normal RBC, no casts	Post-Glomerulo, work up involves CT or cystoscopy or both
Lots of blood, no RBCs	Rhabdomyolysis
Hematuria and blunt trauma	CT scan with IV contrast

CRYPTORCHIDISM	
Path:	Undescended testes
Pt:	Absent testes on physical exam
Dx:	Clinical
Tx:	Newborn: If undescended by 6mo, surgically bring down Prepubertal: Surgically tether Postpubertal: Surgically remove
F/u:	Monitor for testicular cancer (↑ 10x risk)

Seizures

ABSENCE	
Path:	Hundreds of brief seizures without post-ictal state
Pt:	"ADHD" symptoms 　　- Trouble in school 　　- Trouble paying attention
Dx:	EEG
Tx:	Ethosuximide
F/u:	Will outgrow eventually

FEBRILE SEIZURE	
Path:	Peak temp / rate of rise (doesn't matter)
Pt:	Five months to Five years First time seizure Fever and a seizure No focal features (simple) Fifteen minutes or less (simple)
Dx:	Clx
Tx:	Treat underlying cause

WEST SYNDROME	
Path:	Unknown
Pt:	Around 6 months old Bilateral Jerking head or extremities NO FEVER
Dx:	Interictal EEG = Hypsarrhythmia
Tx:	ACTH
F/u:	Psychomotor Retardation

LENNOX-GASTAUT	
Path:	Comes from other causes—West, Tuberous Sclerosis, Brain injury of some kid
Pt:	1-7 years old, Recurrent seizures
Dx:	Interictal EEG spike and wave
Tx:	Valproate, Rufinamide
F/u:	Psychomotor and Intellectual Disability

TUBEROUS SCLEROSIS	
Path:	Brain Tubers
Pt:	< 2 years Afebrile Seizures
Dx:	Ash leaf spots on Wood's Lamp CT scan on Tubers
Tx:	Organ specific—think seizures
F/u:	Monitor for organ involvement—brain, eyes, heart, psych

Immunodeficiencies

B CELLS

X-LINKED AGAMMAGLOBULINEMIA OF BRUTON	
Path:	X-Linked A-Ig-enemia ↓ B Cells = Boys
Pt:	Sinopulmonary infections, 6 months
Dx:	CBC = Normal QIg:　　∅ IgA 　　　　∅ IgG 　　　　∅ IgM Flow = ∅ B Cells BTK Gene
Tx:	Schedule IgG . . . BM transplant

CVID	
Path:	Mild XLA
Pt:	Mild XLA in Teenager
Dx:	CBC = Normal QIG: ↓ 2/3 Ig
Tx:	Schedule IgG . . . BM transplant

IGA DEFICIENCY	
Path:	↓ IgA → ↓ Mucosal
Pt:	1. Sinopulmonary + GI Bugs 2. Asx . . .pRBC . . .anaphylaxis
Dx:	CBC = Normal QIG: ↓ IgA, ↑ IgG, ↑ IgM
Tx:	∅
F/u:	Anaphylaxis

HYPER IGM	
Path:	Isotype switching fails
Pt:	Immune ↓, bacterial infections
Dx:	CBC = Normal QIg: ↓ IgA, ↓ IgG. ↑↑↑ IgM
Tx:	∅
F/u:	Anaphylaxis

Immunodeficiencies

PHAGOCYTES

LEUKOCYTE ADHESION DEFICIENCY	
Path:	WBC can't leave blood
Pt:	Toxic but NO PUS Delayed separation of the cord
Tx:	Biopsy

CHRONIC GRANULOMATOUS DISEASE	
Path:	No respiratory burst, Macrophages Eat, but not kill catalase +
Pt:	Staph Abscess
Dx:	** Nitro Blue - ** CBC = ↑ WBC QIG = ↑ IgM, ↑ IgG
Tx:	BMT

T CELLS

DIGEORGE	
Path:	22q11.2 deletion 3rd pharyngeal pouch
Pt:	Wide-Spaced Eyes Low-Set Ears Absent thymic shadow Small Face Fungi + PCP
Dx:	Syndrome: Clinical CBC = ↓ ALC
Tx:	TMP-SMX PPx IVIg bridge Thymic transplant
F/u:	↓ Calcium 2/2 PTH Tetany, Seizures

COMBINED

WISKOTT-ALDRICH	
Path:	X-linked Boys
Pt:	Eczema + ↓ Plt + Normal Infections
Dx:	CBC = ↓ WBC, ↓ plt QIG: ↑ IgA, ↑ IgE
Tx:	Bone Marrow Transplant

ATAXIA-TELANGIECTASIA
Ataxia, Telangiectasia, ↓Immune . . . DNA Repair, Leukemia, Lymphoma

SCID	
Path:	∅ Immune System ∅ Defense No B, No T Adenosine Deaminase
Pt:	MEGA AIDS FROM BIRTH
Dx:	CBC = ↓ WBC QIG: ∅ IgA, ∅ IgM, ∅ IgG
Tx:	Isolate from everything . . . TMP-SMX against PCP . . . BM transplant

COMPLEMENT	
C1-Esterase Def	Angioedema FFP
C5-C9 Mac Attack	Neisseria

Anxiety Disorders

GENERALIZED ANXIETY DISORDER	
Path:	Constant state of worry
Pt:	Worry about most things on most days of most months (≥ 6 months) ≥ 3 Somatic Complaints
Dx:	Clinical
Tx:	PSYCHOTHERAPY, psychotherapy, psychotherapy SSRI or Buspirone adjunct ~~Benzos~~ (only if panic attack)

SOCIAL PHOBIA (SOCIAL ANXIETY DISORDER)	
Path:	Irrational and exaggerated fear related to social performance Egodystonic 6 mo+ duration
Pt:	Anxiety and Avoidance of stimulus Public Speaking or Public Restrooms
Dx:	Clinical
Tx:	Cognitive Behavioral Therapy β-blockers for public speaking

SPECIFIC PHOBIA	
Path:	Irrational and exaggerated learned fear response to a specific trigger Egodystonic 6 mo+ duration
Pt:	Anxiety and Avoidance of stimulus Spiders, heights, clowns, etc.
Dx:	Clinical
Tx:	Cognitive Behavioral Therapy - Desensitization: longer, better - Flooding: faster, not as good Control with SSRI during CBT

PANIC ATTACK		
Path:	Random and unprovoked bouts of intense anxiety without warning	
Pt:	Shortness of Breath Trembling Unsteadiness Depersonalization Excessive heart rate Numbness Tingling Sweating	Palpitations Abdominal distress Nausea Intense fear of losing control/ dying Chest pain
Dx:	Rule out medical disease - ECG + troponins - Asthma - TSH, Toxicology	
Tx:	Abort—Benzodiazepines CBT to abort without meds Control—SSRI	
F/u:	Agoraphobia	

Impulse Control Disorders

INTERMITTENT EXPLOSIVE DISORDER	
Path:	Trigger = Anxiety Violent Act = Relief Response DISPROPORTIONATE to stressor (verbal, physical, etc.)
Pt:	2 times per week in 3 months WITHOUT harm OR 3 times at all in a year WITH harm ♂ >> ♀ ↓ Sxs with ↑ age
Dx:	Clx
Tx:	Drugs = Therapy = Drugs + Therapy (SSRI) (Self-reflection)

THEFT	KLEPTOMANIA
Desire Able to resist	↓ Anxiety Unable to Resist
HAS value Pt CAN'T afford	Has NO value Pt CAN afford

Planned, with help,
  or provoked by
  external stimuli
	UNplanned,
	  WITHOUT help,
	  and not provoked
	  by external stimuli

Used or Kept NO remorse NO guilt	Stashed, gifted, or returned Remorse, guilt

PYROMANIA	
Path:	Setting Fire = Relief or Pleasure
Pt:	More than 1 occasion Fire Setting for ↓ Anxiety, ↑ sexual arousal, or ↑ pleasure ♂ >> ♀
Dx:	r/o Arson
Tx:	∅ . . . incarceration
F/u:	Reaction Formation

ARSON	PYROMANIA
Monetary gain To cause harm or to destroy	↓ Anxiety Sexual arousal Pleasure

KLEPTOMANIA	
Path:	Trigger = Anxiety Theft = Relief

Pt:	Steals things
	   - little to NO value
	   - pt CAN afford
	   - to ↓ anxiety
	   - gifts / hides items
	   - and feels guilt / remorse
	   - impulsively, alone, without
	       external
	   - provocation

Dx:	r/o Petty Theft
Tx:	∅ . . . ~~incarceration~~ SSRI? Therapy?

QUICK TABLES © ONLINEMEDED   105

OCD and Related Disorders

OBSESSIVE COMPULSIVE DISORDER		
Path:	Obsessions = anxiety-PROVOKING thoughts, unwanted and intrusive Compulsions = anxiety-REDUCING actions, behaviors, or mental acts	
Pt:	*Obsessions*	*Compulsions*
	Contamination Symmetry Safety	Cleaning, Washing Order, Counting Lock Checking
	At least one hour per day Causes impairment at school, work, socially	
Dx:	Clx	
Tx:	CBT is best SSRI or Clomipramine (a TCA)	

HOARDING DISORDER		
Path:	OCD about throwing things away	
Pt:	*Obsessions*	*Compulsions*
	Ridding of Possessions	Retaining useless items like trash or trinkets
	Unsafe or cluttered home	
Dx:	Clx	
Tx:	CBT → SSRI	

BODY DYSMORPHIC DISORDER		
Path:	Perceived flaws in physical appearance	
Pt:	*Obsessions*	*Compulsions*
	Symmetry of body Hair, skin, nose Breasts, butt	Appearance Checking Approval Seeking
	Attempt to have multiple surgeries to correct what isn't broken	
Dx:	Clx	
Tx:	CBT → SSRI	
F/u:	DO NOT perform surgery as desired	

MUSCLE DYSMORPHIC DISORDER		
Path:	Perceived flaws in physical appearance	
Pt:	*Obsessions*	*Compulsions*
	Muscle Size	Excessive Exercise Anabolic Steroids
	Roid Rage, Rhabdo (renal failure), Testicular atrophy, "copper disorder"	
Dx:	Clx	
Tx:	CBT → SSRI	

TRICHOTILLOMANIA		
Path:	General Anxiety with Hair pulling	
Pt:	*Obsessions*	*Compulsions*
	None in Particular	Pulling out hair items like trash
	Alopecia with hair in different lengths	
Dx:	r/o fungus (KOH prep) r/o medical cause for alopecia	
Tx:	CBT → SSRI	
F/u:	Small bowel obstruction (trichobezoar)	

PTSD and Related Disorders

POST-TRAUMATIC AND ACUTE STRESS DISORDERS		
Path:	*Stressor*	*Exposure*
	- Actual Death	- Experienced
	- Threat Death	(Self)
	- Combat	- Witnessed
	- Rape	(strangers)
	- Abuse	- Learned (family)
		- Repeated exposure to effects
Pt:	*Disorder*	
	- Intrusion	Nightmares,
	- Neg Mood	Flashbacks,
	- Dissociation	memories
	- Avoidance	Depression-like
	- Arousal	Depersonalization, amnesia
		Symbols, locations, memories
		Hypervigilance, irritability, easily startled, CHANGED concentration
Dx:	> 3 days AND < 1 month = Acute Stress	
	> 1 month = Post-Traumatic Stress	
Tx:	Group Therapy (best)	
	SSRI/SNRI (adjunct)	
	~~Benzos~~ (panic attack only)	
	CBT	
F/u:	Mood disorder	
	Substance abuse disorder	

ADJUSTMENT DISORDER	
Path:	Stressor = Non-life-threatening event - Marital strife, loss of a job, moving away
Pt:	Disorder = Mood changes that don't quite fit for another mood disorder
Dx:	Begin < 3 months from stressor Lasts < 6 months from stressors
Tx:	Generally not needed

RAD / DESD	
Path:	Stressor = Neglect or Abuse in infancy
Pt:	Disorder = too much attachment (DSED) too little attachment (RAD)
Dx:	< 5 years old r/o Autism
Tx:	Caregiver—teach how to parent
F/u:	Mood disorder Learning disabilities

Mood Disorders

MAJOR DEPRESSIVE DISORDER	
Path:	↓ mood OR Anhedonia And Duration ≥ 2 weeks AND 5 of SIG-E-CAPS

Pt:	Sleep	↓	↑
	Interest	↓	↓
	Guilt	↑	↑
	Energy	↓	↓
	Concentration	↓	↓
	Appetite	↓	↑
	Psychomotor	↓	↓
	Suicidal	↑	↑

Dx:	r/o Suicidal Ideations
Tx:	If + SI + Plan → Hospital If + SI, NO Plan → Safety Contract Combo >> SSRI /SNRI > Psycho Therapy ECT best (refractory only)

BIPOLAR I	
Path:	Mania = "E" + 3 Duration ≥ 1 week

Pt:	**D**istractibility **F**light of Ideas
	Insomnia **A**gitation
	Grandiosity **S**exual Exploits
	    Talkative
	    Elevated Mood
	    Racing Thoughts

Dx:	r/o Bipolar II r/o Cyclothymia

Tx:	Emergency department = Benzos
	Mood stabilizers = Lithium >
	   Valproate backup = Lamotrigine,
	   Carbamazepine
	Anti-Psychotics = Quetiapine

BIPOLAR II	
Path:	Hypomania AND major depression
Pt:	Hypomania = mania, but less
Dx:	r/o Bipolar I (catatonia, psychotic)
Tx:	Bipolar I
F/u:	If Major Depression, started SSRI, then have Mania → reveals Bipolar I

DYSTHYMIA = PERSISTENT DEPRESSIVE DISORDER	
Pt:	↓ Mood for ≥ 2 years Symptoms ∅ absent 2+ months
Dx:	r/o hypothyroid
Tx:	SSRI / SNRI

CYCLOTHYMIA	
Pt:	Mild Bipolar II

Mood II Life and Death

	BABY BLUES	POST-PARTUM DEPRESSION	POST-PARTUM PSYCHOSIS
Baby	# 1 Cares about baby	> #1 Doesn't care about baby, may hurt baby	> # 1 Fears the baby, likely to kill it
Timing	Onset and Duration within 2 weeks	Onset within 1 month Duration ongoing	Onset within 1 month Duration ongoing
Depression	Dysthymic	MDE	MDE
Psychosis	None	None	⊕
Treatment	Nothing	Anti-depressants	Mood Stabilizers or Antipsychotics

	GRIEF	PCBD	DEPRESSION
Onset	Any	≥ 6 months	Any
Duration	< 12 months	≥ 12 months	≥ 12 months
Focus - Dysphoria - Guilt - Anhedonia	Focused on Deceased	Focused on Deceased	Pervasive, global
When mood symptoms	Waxes, wanes, can imagine happy	Persistent ⊕ Cannot imagine being happy	Persistent ⊕ Cannot imagine being happy
Behaviors	YES insight "Psychotic" Talking TO deceased Doing things as if they were there	NO Insight Psychotic features	NO Insight Psychotic - Hallucinations - Delusions Talking WITH deceased Believing they are there doing things with you
Why suicide	To be with deceased		To end suffering, despondent
Treatment	Time, Counseling	SSRI	SSRI

STAGES OF DEATH AND DYING
Denial
Depression
Bargaining
Anger
Acceptance

Psychotic Disorders

DELUSIONS
Fixed False Belief without basis in reality
Do NOT confront delusion; it is a glaring truth to the patient, and you will not get anywhere by challenging them.

SCHIZOPHRENIA	
Path:	Thought Disorder with unknown cause though there is certainly a genetic component Receptor Pathology - Dopamine (too much) → + Sxs - Serotonin (too much) → - Sxs
Pt:	**Psychotic Break** = first break occurs in teenager with stressor (college) who then begins behaving bizarrely **Positive Symptoms (must have 1+)** - Bizarre Delusions - Hallucinations, usually auditory (voices) - Disorganized speech - Disorganized state / catatonia **Negative Symptoms:** - Anhedonia - Flat Affect - Cognitive Defects
Dx:	Clinical r/o drug abuse (cocaine)
Tx:	Anti-psychotics - Typical controls positive symptoms - Atypical controls negative symptoms - Clozapine when all else fails

VARIANTS AND DURATION OF TREATMENT		
All variants have the exact same pathology, sxs, presentation, and diagnosis, EXCEPT the time those symptoms have been present. This leads to duration of treatment with anti-psychotics		
	Duration Sxs	*Duration Tx*
Acute Psychotic Disorder	< 1 Month	Wait (or treat)
Schizophreniform	< 6 Months	3-6 weeks
Schizophrenia	≥ 6 Months	Lifetime
Schizoaffective	Any with mood sxs	Lifetime treat delusion first

TREATMENT OPTIONS FOR PSYCHOTIC DISORDERS		
⊕ Sxs	Typical	Haloperidol, Thiazide, Chlorpromazine
⊖ Sxs	Atypical	Risperidone, Quetiapine, Olanzapine, Ziprasidone, Aripiprazole
Best		Clozapine

Eating Disorders

ANOREXIA NERVOSA	
Path:	Anxiety induced by the fear of being or becoming fat Patient is not fat, but fears fat; sees herself as fat Lacks recognition of how thin she is

Pt:	F:M 10:1, teens to 20s
	Severe
	   - hypotension, bradycardia, leukopenia
	   - CMP abnormalities, E-lytes and albumin
	   - BMI < 16
	Non-Severe
	   - Lanugo, Cold-intolerance, Amenorrhea, Emaciation

Dx:	Clx

Tx:	Hospitalize if severe
	   - IV Nutrition
	   - Correct E-Lytes
	   - Forced Feed
	Outpatient / ongoing
	   - Antipsychotics and CBT

F/u:	If OCD or MDD, add SSRI / SnRI Relapse in 5 years Death from medical or suicide

METHODS OF EATING DISORDERS	
Restriction	↓ Caloric intake (fasting, dieting) ↑ Caloric expenditure (exercise)
Binge Purge Emesis	Eating / Binging then induced emesis Dorsal hand scars (from emesis) Dental erosion (from emesis) Metabolic Alkalosis, K, Mg disorders
Binge Purge Laxative	Eating / Binging then induced diarrhea Metabolic Acidosis Diarrhea

BULIMIA NERVOSA	
Path:	Anxiety from the binge, then compensates Normal weight to overweight
Pt:	F:M 10:1, teens to 20s "normal" appearance except purge signs Purge ≥ 1 x per week x 3 months
Dx:	Clx
Tx:	SSRI / SnRI = Fluoxetine (best) CBT
F/u:	NEVER Bupropion (causes seizures)

BINGE-EATING DISORDER	
Path:	Anxiety from the binge—no compensation Overweight to obese
Pt:	F:M 10:1, teens to 20s Cannot control eating habits Binge ≥ 1 x per week x 3 months
Dx:	Clx
Tx:	Topiramate CBT

Personality Disorders

	PD	DESCRIPTION	EXAMPLES	HOW TO HANDLE THEM
A	Paranoid	**Distrustful, suspicious,** interpret others are malicious	*"Enemy of the State"* Gene Hackman,	Clear, honest, nonthreatening
	Schizoid	Loners, have no relationships but also are **happy not having any relationships**	Night-Shift Toll Booth	You won't see them
	Schizotypal	**Magical Thinking,** borders on psychosis, Bizarre Thoughts, Behavior, and Dress	Lady Gaga	Brief Psychotic Episodes Clear, honest, nonthreatening
B	Borderline	Unstable, Impulsive, Promiscuous, emotional emptiness, unable to control **rapid changes in mood, suicidal gestures**	*"Girl Interrupted"* *"Fatal Attraction"*	Suicidal Gestures may be successful **Splitting, Dialectical Behavioral Therapy**
	Histrionic	**Theatrical,** attention-seeking, hypersexual, **use of physical appearance,** dramatic, Exaggerated but superfluous emotions	*"Gone with the Wind"* Marilyn Monroe	Set rules, insist they are followed
	Narcissistic	**Inflated sense of worth** or talent, self-centered, fragile ego, uses eccentric dress to draw attention, **demands special treatment**	*"Zoolander"* Ron Burgundy	Set rules, insist they are followed
	Anti-Social	**Criminal.** No regards for rights of others, impulsive, **lacks remorse,** manipulative. Must be **>18 years old** (conduct disorder)	Tony Soprano The Joker	**Jail,** Set rules, insist they are followed
C	Avoidant	Fears rejection and criticism, **wants relationships** but **does not pursue** them, Passes on promotions	*"Napoleon Dynamite"* Shy hot librarian	Avoid power struggles, make patients choose
	Dependent	Unable to assume responsibility. Submissive, clingy, **fears being alone**	Stay at home mom in an abusive relationship	Give clear advice, patient may try to sabotage their own treatment
	Obsessive-Compulsive	Rigid, orderly perfectionist. Order, Control. Perfection at the expense of efficacy	*"Monk"*	

Dissociative Disorders

DISSOCIATIVE DISORDERS IN GENERAL	
Path:	Severe + Prolonged Stressor causes separation of otherwise intact thought, memory, and identity
Pt:	Stressor proportional to Disorder
Dx:	Amytal Interview (truth serum) r/o malingering r/o substance abuse
Tx:	Psychotherapy
F/u:	Non-severe = recovery Severe =?

DEPERSONALIZATION DEREALIZATION DISORDER	
Path:	Adolescent with minor stressor (though stressor is relatively major for demographic)
Pt:	Seeing a video or dream of self, out-of-body experience (depersonalization) Detached from reality, as though in a dream Reality testing INTACT

DISSOCIATIVE IDENTITY DISORDER	
Path:	≥ 2 distinct identity states Most severe and prolonged trauma
Pt:	Self experiences - Memory gaps (blackouts) - other dissociation symptoms Others Witness - Paradoxical behaviors - Appearance changes
F/u:	*Fight Club, Sybil*

DISSOCIATIVE AMNESIA	
Path:	Stressors induce loss of memory
Pt:	Memory Loss of - the event - regular everyday occurrences / routine - complete autobiographical self
F/u:	*Law and Order, SVU*

DISSOCIATIVE AMNESIA WITH FUGUE	
Path:	Stressors induce loss of memory WITH Travel
Pt:	Memory Loss of - the event - regular everyday occurrences / routine - complete autobiographical self
F/u:	*Jason Bourne, Archer from FX*

PSYCH

Catatonia

CATATONIA	

Path:	∅ a disease state
	Modifier to another disease
	   ψ—Bipolar, Depression >> schizophrenia
	   ♥—Autoimmune, paraneoplastic, nutritional

Pt:	Must have 3 or more:
	  - Stupor
	  - Cata-LEPSY
	  - Waxy flexibility Retarded
	  - Mutism Catatonia
	  - Negativism
	
	  - Stereotypy
	  - Agitation or Grimace Excited
	  - Echolalia Catatonia
	  - Echopraxia
	
	Retarded and Excited symptoms may
	  occur together

Dx:	Clx . . . Lorazepam
Tx:	Lorazepam (diagnostic and therapeutic)

Dz	Meds / Hx	Sxs
Malignant Catatonia	No meds, lorazepam corrects	Rigidity Autonomic Dysfunction (↑ BP, ↑ HR, ↑ T)
Neuroleptic Malignant Hyperthermia	Atypical Antipsychotics Lead-Pipe Rigidity	Muscle breakdown ("↑ CK")
Serotonin Syndrome	SSRIs and Hypertonicity/ Hyperreflexia	
Malignant Hyperthermia	Halothane anesthesia, family history	

Peds: Neurodevelopmental

INTELLECTUAL DISABILITY DISORDER	

Path:	Chromosomal:
	   - Down Syndrome
	   - Fragile X
	   - Cri-Du-Chat
	Maternal Acquired
	   - EtOH in utero
	   - Hypothyroid in utero
	Child Acquired
	   - Lead Poisoning
	   - Head Trauma

Pt:	↓ Cognitive skill ↓ Adaptive Functioning +/- Syndromic physical features
Dx:	Clx; severity on adaptive functioning Severity based on IQ testing (outdated)
Tx:	Assess social, conceptual (speak, read write), and practical (self mgmt) Special education, supervision
	50-70 Group home, Work and ADLs alone
	35-49 Group home, Work and ADLs alone
	20-34 Institutionalized, Supervised ADLs
	< 20 Institutionalized, Total Care

TIC DISORDER (TOURETTE'S)	
Path:	Essentially OCD

Pt:	Onset < 18 years old
	"Obsession" = impulse to perform tic
	"Compulsion" = the tic itself
	   Hidden: hair flicks, blinking, rubbing
	   Vocal: Grunt, cough, yell
	   NEVER a swear word

Dx:	Clx
Tx:	Dopamine Antagonists - Fluphenazine, Tetrabenazine
F/u:	ADHD on stimulants who gets worse is Tic Disorder

AUTISM SPECTRUM	

Path:	**Impaired Social Communication**
	   - Social Reciprocity
	   - Social Relationships
	   - Nonverbal Communication
	   - Joint Attending
	Restrictive / Repetitive Behavior
	   - Stereotypy
	   - Sameness
	   - Restricted Interests
	   - Change in perception

Pt:	Young child, 1-4 years old No social smile or eye contact Repetitive useless behaviors Insistence on consistency
Dx:	Clx; Severity based on progress
Tx:	Supportive
F/u:	NO ASSOCIATION WITH VACCINES

ATTENTION DEFICIT HYPERACTIVITY DISORDER	

Path:	**Impulsivity**
	   - Blurts out answers
	   - Interrupts
	   - Fidgets a lot
	   - Cannot wait turn
	Inattention
	   - Talks Fast
	   - Easily Distracted
	   - Fails to complete tasks
	Timing and situation
	   - ≥ 2 settings
	   - onset 7-12
	   - duration ≥ 6 months

Pt:	The "bad kid" who is male, disrupts class and moves all over the place, fails to wait his turn, whose parents have a tough time controlling behaviorally, and who's like this in every setting. Ensure there are no absence seizures
Dx:	Clx

Tx:	Stimulants (avoid at night to ↓ insomnia)
	   - Methylphenidate
	   - Dextroamphetamine

F/u:	Special ed classes, parent education If absence seizures, carbamazepine

Peds: Neurodevelopmental

	LEARNING DISABILITIES
Path:	Performing substantially below expected for age and grade

Pt:	Medical Conditions
	  - Deaf, Blind, Non-native Speaker
	Poor Education to Date
	  - Low socioeconomic class, home schooled

Dx:	Audiology test Vision testing Language assessment
Tx:	Remediate, fix the medical problem (glasses, hearing aids), fix the teacher to student ratio

Peds: Behavioral

CONDUCT DISORDER	
Path:	Antisocial personality disorder but ... < 18 years old

Pt:	**Bullying**
	   - Hurts animals / people
	   - Uses torture / cruelty
	   - Forced Sex
	Destruction
	   - Fire starting
	   - Lies, Cheats, Steal
	   - Breaks into property
	Rules Violation
	   - Truancy
	   - Run-away at least twice
	   - Staying out at night before 13

Dx:	Clx
Tx:	Juvenile Detention
F/u:	Fights Authority HARMS peers

OPPOSITIONAL DEFIANT DISORDER	
Path:	Incongruent parenting Teen acting out

Pt:	**NO Bullying**
	   - Does NOT hurt animals / people
	   - Does NOT use torture / cruelty
	   - Forced Sex
	Destruction
	   - Lies, Cheats, Steal
	   - Breaks into property
	Rules Violation
	   - Truancy
	   - Run-away at least twice
	   - Staying out at night before 13

Dx:	Clx
Tx:	Improved Parenting
F/u:	Fights Authority COOPERATES with peers

ENURESIS—NEVER BEEN DRY	
Path:	Normal toilet training takes up to 7 years old
Pt:	If < 7 and still wets bed, it's NORMAL
Dx:	Clx
Tx:	POSITIVE reinforcement Alarm Blankets Water Restriction before bed DDAVP as last resort
F/u:	TCAs may also be used ~~Negative Reinforcement~~ (never)

ENURESIS—WAS ONCE DRY	
Path:	Regression, Abuse, Infection, Anatomic
Pt:	Was once dry, now is not
Dx:	U/A U/S Clx
Tx:	Infection (abx); if STI then abuse Anatomic (resection) Regression (identify stressor); abuse

ENCOPRESIS AND ENURESIS	

Path:	Encopresis (stool) or Enuresis (urine) repeatedly on clothes or bed.
	   - Intentional (acting out)
	   - Incontinent(cognitive impairment)
	   - Medication side effect
	   - Anatomic (fistula)
	   - Regression (abuse, stressor)

Pt:	Dependent on patients. Look for new sibling, new step parent, or new house
Dx:	See above
Tx:	See above

Pharmacology I: Anti-Depressants + Mood Stabilizers

ANTI-DEPRESSANTS		
SSRIs	(Es)citalopram Fluoxetine Paroxetine Sertraline	↓ **Libido** sometimes **Delayed Ejaculation** sometimes Serotonin Syndrome GI, Insomnia
SnRIs	(Des)Venlafaxine Duloxetine	Cleaner, better versions of SSRIs. More expensive
Atypical	Bupropion	**Smoking cessation** No weight gain ~~Bulimia~~ NEVER (↑ seizures)
SM	Mirtazapine Trazadone	Appetite Stimulant Sleep Aid, caution priapism
TCAs	"-triptylines" Imipramine Desipramine Doxepin	Used for **enuresis** (anti-ACh) 1st line use is **neuropathic pain** Can be **Lethal** because of CCC: (Convulsions, Coma, Cardiac) so get an ECG Has **Anti-ACh** properties (dry mouth, sedation, urinary retention, constipation)
MAO-Is	Phenelzine Tranylcypromine Selegiline	**HTN Crisis** when mixed together, lack of washout or eating of **tyramine** (red wine/cheese) Distinguish from other hypertensive-hyperthermia disorders in psych by the ABSENCE of lead-pipe rigidity and fever

MOOD STABILIZERS		
Drug	*Indication*	*Side Effect*
Lithium	**First-Line, Drug of Choice** for Bipolar Bipolar, Acute Mania, Depression Augmentation	**Teratogen** **Nephrotoxic > 1.5** Causes Nephro DI Narrow TI
Valproate	**First Line** in Bipolar if Li cannot be used Also treats Seizures	**Teratogen** (Spina Bifida) Thrombocytopenia Agranulocytosis Pancreatitis
Quetiapine	**Second Line** bipolar All phases of treatment	Weight gain QTc prolongation
Lamotrigine	**Second Line** bipolar Newer anticonvulsant	Blurred Vision SJS
Carbamazepine	Third line bipolar Trigeminal Neuralgia Absence Seizures	**Teratogen** (Cleft palate) Rash, SJS AV Block

ANTI-ANXIETY		
Benzos	**Abort** panic attack Treats **EtOH** withdrawal	**Dependence** **Withdrawal Seizure**
SSRIs	**First-Line** long term medication for treatment of chronic anxiety: OCD, PTSD, GAD	See Anti-Depressants. ∅ useful in acute attack
β-Blockers	**Performance Anxiety**	Bradycardia, Asthma

Pharmacology II: Anti-Anxiety + Anti-Psychotics

ANTIPSYCHOTICS		
Typicals = First Generation Antispsychotics (FGA)		

Haloperidol
Fluphenazine
Thioridazine
Chlorpromazine
	Mesolimbic D2C-R-i
	  treats ⊕ symptoms
		Potency of drug proportional
		  to EPS

	Nigrostriatal Antagonism leads to EPS side
	  effects
		Potency inversely
		  proportional to Anti-ACh

	Tuberoinfundibular antagonism causes ↑ prolactin, gynecomastia	
Atypicals = Second generation Antipsychotics (SGA)		

Risperidone
Quetiapine
Olanzapine
Aripiprazole
Ziprasidone
	Both **D2$_C$** and **5-HT$_1$** so
	  work on ⊕ and ⊖ sxs
	More selective so lower risk of EPS
	Currently "first line" for psychosis
		QTc prolongation
		EPS, Gynecomastia,
		  Sedation, Anti-ACh
		  (small risk)
		DM and **Weight Gain**

Clozapine		
Unique to itself	The **best antipsychotic** The most selective for **D2$_C$** and **5HT$_1$** (and) Drug of **last resort**	**Agranulocytosis** Requiring CBC q week

EXTRAPYRAMIDAL SIDE EFFECTS		
Akathisia	A **Feeling of Restlessness**	↓Dose . . .. β-blockers Anti-ACh (Benztropine)
Acute Dystonia	Involuntary muscle contractions, hand ringing, torticollis, and **oculogyric crisis**	Anti-ACh (Benztropine)
Dyskinesia	**Parkinsonism** Dyskinesia = Bradykinesia	Anti-ACh (Benztropine)

Tardive Dyskinesia	Irreversible **hypersensitization** of
	  dopamine-R = suppressible
	  oral-facial movements
		Stop Drug,
		Sxs **initially worsen**

CHOOSING THE RIGHT DRUG		
Compliant Young Adult, without complications	Any atypical po	↓ SE profile
Combative ER patient	Haloperidol Depot	Sedating
Noncompliant Psychotic	Olanzapine depot Risperidone depot Haloperidol depot	q 1wk
Dysphagia or IM not available	Olanzapine ODT Risperidone ODT	Oral dissolving tablet
Everything else has failed	**Clozapine**	Best, most dangerous
Hospitalized and off their meds	Atypical, ↑ **Dose q Day** until maxed, then try another	

Addiction I: Substance Abuse

SUBSTANCE ABUSE DISORDER		
Path:	Using a drug or alcohol in any other way than it is intended Substance = Drug, Alcohol, gambling, sex	
Pt:	Difficulty Controlling Use	1. Consuming more than was intended 2. Difficulty cutting down or stopping 3. Investing time in obtaining of recovering from use 4. Craving
	Adverse Social Outcomes	5. Failure of responsibilities at work, home, school 6. Choosing substance over people relationships 7. Giving up what you used to like to do
	Risk Taking	8. Use in hazardous condition (legal issues, sex, driving) 9. Use despite previous consequences
	Health Effects	10. Tolerance: needing more to feel the same effect 11. Withdrawal: physical symptoms when stopped
Dx:	Severity	Mild 2-3 Moderate 4-5 Severe 6+
	Screen CAGE	**C**ut down **A**nger about criticism **G**uilt about using or what you do when using **E**ye-opener
Tx:	Pharm	Antabuse (disulfiram for EtOH) Naloxone (Opiate, EtOH) Methadone (Opiates) Usually pharm doesn't work
	Group Therapy	Alcoholics Anonymous
F/u:	50-90% will relapse Relapse is not failure Back on the horse	
	F Feedback	
	R Responsibility—sobriety and mistakes	
	A Advice—help them	
	M Menu of options	
	E Empathy	
	S Self-Efficacy	

FIVE STAGES OF SUBSTANCE ABUSE	
Pre-contemplative	Unaware, denial
Contemplative	Admits there's a problem, acceptance
Preparation	Committed, taking steps
Action	Actual changing behavior
Maintenance	Sustained changed behavior

Addiction II: Drugs of Abuse

DRUG	INTOXICATION	WITHDRAWAL	DRUG / ANTIDOTE
EtOH	Slurred speech, Disinhibition, Ataxia, Blackouts, Memory Loss, Impaired Judgment	Tachycardia and HTN, Tremor, perspiration, hallucinations, and eventual seizures	**Benzo Taper** (withdrawal) **Disulfiram** (Long-Term)
Benzos	Delirium in elderly, **Respiratory Depression** and **coma** (with ↑ dose), amnesia	Tremor, **Tachycardia,** HTN, **Seizures,** Psychosis	**Flumazenil**
Opiates	Euphoria, **pupil constriction, respiratory depression**, and potential **track marks**	**Yawning**, lacrimation, N/V and hurts everywhere, sweating	**Naloxone** **Methadone** (long-term)
Cocaine	Psychomotor agitation, **HTN, tachycardia, dilated pupils, psychosis** **Angina / HTN** crisis	Depression, suicidality, irritability, "cocaine bugs"	Supportive Care Benzos / antipsychotics for agitation HTN treated with α then β blockade
MDMA	**Overheat** (fever, tachycardia) and **water intoxication**. Pupillary Dilation, Psychosis	Crash	Supportive
PCP	**Aggressive** psychosis, **vertical, lateral,** or **rotary nystagmus,** impossible strength, blunted senses	Severe random Violence	Haloperidol to subdue **Acidify Urine** to enhance excretion
LSD	Hallucinations, Flashbacks, Heightened senses, dissociative symptoms	Flashbacks	Supportive
THC	Tiredness, slowed reflexes, **conjunctivitis**, the **munchies**, overdose brings **paranoia**	∅	Supportive (often nothing required)
Barbs	Low safety margins, Benzos safer	Redistribute into fat	∅
Nicotine	None—just jittery and stimulated. Pt has to Overdose a lot → VFib	Cravings	**Bupropion** Chantix (Varenicline)
Amphetamines	Tachycardia, hypertension, pressured speech, flight of ideas	Crash	**None**

Sleep I: Physiology

STAGE	EEG
Awake	State of arousal
N I	Theta Waves, Absence of Alpha
N II	K-Komplexes, Sleep Spindles
N III	δ waves
REM	Awake EEG, Atony, Saccadic Eyes, Erections

SLEEP WALKING / EATING/ DRIVING / SEX	
Path:	N3 Sleep Stage
Pt:	Do actions without remembering
Dx:	Clx
Tx:	Reassurance
F/u:	Worse with BZD_1 (zolpidem)

VOCABULARY OF SLEEP	
Sleep Latency	Going to bed to falling asleep ↑ in insomnia ↓ in sleep deprivation
REM Latency	Falling asleep (N1) to REM ↓ in Narcolepsy ↓ in sleep deprivation
REM Rebound	More REM faster after Deprivation state

NIGHT TERROR	
Path:	N3 Sleep Stage
Pt:	Child 4-10 who will: - maintain tone, sit up, opens eyes - be asleep (inconsolable) - not remember anything Parents distressed, kids aren't
Dx:	Clx
Tx:	Reassurance

NIGHTMARE	
Path:	Dreams gone bad, REM
Pt:	Any age group wakens from sleep, remembers the dream
Dx:	Clx
Tx:	Treat underlying psych condition (PTSD) If not part of syndrome, no need to treat

SLEEP TALKING	
Path:	N3 Sleep Stage
Pt:	Mumbling in sleep Will not reveal secrets
Dx:	Clx
Tx:	Reassurance

Sleep II: Disorders

OBSTRUCTIVE SLEEP APNEA	
Path:	Excess tissue of oropharynx and chest wall (obesity) obstructs airway Multiple awakenings prevent progression to REM Ventilation spared (CO_2 normal) Oxygenation impaired ($\downarrow O_2$)
Pt:	Obese, snores, short neck, difficult to exam oropharynx Daytime Somnolence ("sleeps" but never reaches REM, so not restful sleep) Cor Pulmonale
Dx:	Polysomnography (Sleep Study) - 15 apneas / hour - 5 apneas / hr + snoring
Tx:	CPAP = PEEP Weight loss
F/u:	$\downarrow$ Alveolar Oxygen → Pulm Htn Pulm htn = isolated heart failure.

NARCOLEPSY	
Path:	Uncertain Etiology
Pt:	"Sleep Attack" . . . wakes REFRESHED - Cataplexy, Paralysis - $\downarrow$ REM Latency - HypoGOgic / Hypnopompic - Response to emotion or bang - Wakeup Refreshed 3 times per week x 3 months
Dx:	CSF Hypocretin 1 (Also polysomnography)
Tx:	Scheduled Naps Stimulants (Amphetamines)

INSOMNIA	
Path:	Poor sleep hygiene For this setting, assume no psych illness
Pt:	Trouble falling asleep Trouble staying asleep < 6 hrs / night total sleep
Dx:	r/o MDD . . . SIGECAPS r/o Bipolar . . . DIGFASTER r/o substance . . . caffeine, cocaine
Tx:	Lifestyle = Sleep Hygiene - Avoid stimulants w/i 5 hrs of sleep - Avoid exercise near sleep - Avoid naps during the day - Bed for sex and sleep only - Lights Out = Sleep Time Pharm - Diphenhydramine → Trazadone → Quetiapine → Zolpidem

JET LAG
Insomnia and Travel
Power through and Melatonin

CENTRAL SLEEP APNEA
Patient "forgets" to breathe
$\downarrow$ Ventilation = $\uparrow CO_2$ = Altered, Acidotic
Caused by opiates, stroke. Has Cheyne-Stokes

Gender Dysphoria

GENDER TERMS	
Assignment	Your Genitals at birth "What you are physically"
Gender Identity	Your gender in your mind "What you are mentally"
Transgender	Someone who's identity is more often incongruent than their assignment
Transsexual	Not only identifying, but has socially or physically changed to another assignment
Transvestic Disorder	Cross-Dressing but NOT transgendered

GENDER DYSPHORIA	
Path:	Assignment DOES-NOT-EQUAL Identity AND Distress over incongruence
Pt:	6-month duration AND any 1 of: - Assignment DOES-NOT-EQUAL Identity - desire to BE, or to be TREATED as dif gender - Wanting to rid sex char - Belief that they are another gender KIDS - Add REJECT roles of assignment - Add ACCEPT roles of opposite
Dx:	Clx
Tx:	Therapy >> surgery reassignment and hormones

DEFINING PARAPHILIAS	
Common	
Pedophilia	Sexual focus on children Often Male adult → female child
Exhibitionism	Exposing genitals to strangers
Voyeurism	Observing private activities of unaware victims
Frotteurism	Touching, rubbing or a nonconsenting person
Uncommon	
Fetishism	Inanimate objects
Masochism	Being humiliated or forced to suffer
Sadism	Inflicting humiliation or pain on others
Transvestic disorder	Sexually aroused by cross dressing

Somatic Symptom Disorder

SOMATIC SYMPTOM DISORDER (NEW SOMATIZATION)	
Path:	Somatic anxiety disorder with or without explanation
Pt:	≥ 6 months AND One or more somatic symptoms OR - High level of Health related anxiety - Disproportionate concern to seriousness - Excessive time and energy devoted to them
Tx:	Psychotherapy

CONVERSION DISORDER	
Path:	Life Stressor NOT intentional NOT fabricated
Pt:	Sensory or Motor Related to the Stressor La belle Indifference Will not harm self
Tx:	Psychotherapy Confront Stressor

ILLNESS ANXIETY DISORDER (HYPOCHONDRIASIS)	
Pt:	Preoccupation with GETTING SICK Usually has no illness or complaint
Dx:	r/o organic disease
Tx:	One provider, set limits—do not over test Psychotherapy

FACTITIOUS / MUNCHAUSEN'S	
Pt:	Conscious, intentional fabrication to play the sick role Grid-Iron Abdomen Flight at Confrontation Abuse of a dependent (By Proxy)
Tx:	Confrontation of Factitious Jail of Factitious by proxy

MALINGERING	
Pt:	Conscious, intentional fabrication to obtain secondary gain Get money (disability), get drugs (ED, UC), get freedom (out of jail)
Tx:	Confrontation

Gynecologic Cancers

CERVICAL CANCER	
Path:	HPV infection → 16, 18, 30s
Pt:	Asx screen = Pap (pre-cancer) Post-Coital Bleeding Reproductive Aged Female

Dx:	Pap Smear
	   - Start screen at 21, then q3y
	   - ASCUS: q1y Pap or HPV
	      DNA
	Colposcopy
	   - Ectocervical lesions
	   - Endocervical lesions
	Staging

Tx:	Ecto: local ablation (Leep, Cryo) Endo: cone biopsy Stage IIa or < : Local resection Stage IIb or > : Chemo + Radiation
Screen:	Pap Smear

Prevent:	HPV Vaccine
	   - Girls 11-26
	   - Boys 11-21

ENDOMETRIAL CANCER	

Path:	Progesterone is Protective
	Estrogen exposure
	   - Old age
	   - Nulliparity
	   - Obesity
	   - PCOS
	   - Hormone Replacement Therapy

Pt:	Post-menopausal female with post- menopausal bleeding
Dx:	Endometrial Sampling or D+C (Biopsy)

Tx:	Hyperplasia: Progesterone
	Cancer: TAH + BSO
	   +/- Radiation
	   +/- Chemo

VULVAR CANCER	
Path:	Squamous Cell (HPV) Melanoma (Sun Exposure)
Pt:	Black and Itchy
Dx:	1st and Best = Biopsy
Tx:	Vulvectomy and LN Dissection

PAGET'S	
Path:	Usually non-invasive
Pt:	RED and Itchy
Dx:	1st and Best = Biopsy
Tx:	Local resection (no need for vulvectomy)

GERM CELL OVARIAN CANCER	
Subtypes:	Dysgerminomas: Chemo, LDH Endometrial Sinus: AFP Teratoma: Struma Ovarii Chorio: β-hCG
Path:	Nonmalignant
Pt:	Teenage girl with an adnexal mass Stage I
Dx:	Transvaginal Ultrasound Best: Biopsy
Tx:	Unilateral Salpingo- Oopherectomy (conservative)

EPITHELIAL CELL OVARIAN CANCER	
Subtypes:	Serous Mucinous Endometrioid Brenner's
Path:	Epithelial Trauma = Ovulation Malignant

Pt:	Post-menopausal female
	Null/Low Parity
	Stage IIIb or worse (even
	   with screen)
	   - Asx, seed peritoneally
	   - Renal Failure, SBO,
	      Ascites
	BRCA 1 or 2, HNPCC

Dx:	NO screen 1st: Transvaginal Ultrasound Then: CT –stage Track: Ca-125 Best: Biopsy
Tx:	TAH + BSO Paclitaxel

Special:	BRCA1 or 2 screen
	   Transvaginal U/S and Ca-
	   125 with PPx TAH+BSO
	   @ 35

Gynecologic Cancers

STROMAL CELL OVARIAN TUMORS	
Path:	Granulosa Theca—Estrogen Sertoli-Leydig—Testosterone

VAGINAL CANCER	
SCC	Just like Cervical cancer except no pap
Adeno	DES exposure in mom while your patient in front of you was in mom's uterus. "Grape-Like" mass in vagina in a child

Gestational Trophoblastic

COMPLETE MOLE	
Path:	Completely Molar = No Fetal Parts Completely Chromosomal = 46,XX Completely Spermal = No egg genetics Normal Fertilization Broken Egg
Pt:	Size-Date Discrepancy β-hCG too high for dates Hyperthyroidism (from β-hCG) Hyperemesis Gravidarum Adnexal mass (simple cyst) Grape-like mass exiting cervix
Dx:	1st: U/S Snowstorm ****
Tx:	Suction Curettage
F/u:	β-hCG q week OCP x 1 year

INCOMPLETE MOLE	
Path:	Incompletely Molar = Some Fetal Parts Incompletely Chromosomal = t69, XXY Abnormal Fertilization = 2 sperm Normal Egg
Pt:	Size-Date discrepancy β-hCG too high for dates Hyperthyroidism (from β-hCG) Hyperemesis Gravidarum Adnexal mass (simple cyst) Grape-like mass exiting cervix
Dx:	1st: U/S Snowstorm ****
Tx:	Suction Curettage
F/u:	β-hCG q week OCP x 1 year

CHORIOCARCINOMA	
Path:	Cancer of gestational contents
Pt:	s/p Mole, Miscarriage, or even normal pregnancy ↑ β-hCG (sxs as above)
Dx:	1st: transvaginal ultrasound Best: Biopsy = Curettage Then: Stage CT

Tx:	Surgical
	   - TAH (I)
	   - Debulking (III)
	Medical = "MAC"
	   - Methotrexate
	   - Actinomycin D
	   - Cyclophosphamide
	Chemo = "MAC Backbone"
	   - Advanced only

GYN

Incontinence

STRESS INCONTINENCE	
Path:	Big / Multiple Births Stretch Cardinal Ligament Cystocele Abd pressure on = bladder, not sphincter
Pt:	Sneeze and pee ⊘ Urge ⊘ Nocturnal sxs
Dx:	Physical = Cystocele <s>U/A</s> <s>Cystometry</s> Q-Tip Test
Tx:	1st Lifestyle Then PT, Pessaries Then Surgery (sling / urethral bulking agents)

IRRITATIVE BLADDER	
Path:	Inflammation Stones, UTIs, Cancer
Pt:	Frequency, Urgency, Dysuria + Urge ⊘ nocturnal symptoms
Dx:	Physical = Normal U/A = Dx → Urine Cx <s>Cystometry</s>
Tx:	UTI: FQ, Bactrim, Nitrofurantoin
F/u:	Stones and Cancer (Urology, Medicine)

HYPERTONIC BLADDER / MOTOR URGE	
Path:	Spastic contractions Random detrusor contractions
Pt:	+ Urge + Nocturnal Sxs Pee when spasms
Dx:	Physical = Normal U/A = Normal Cystometry = Spasms at all urinary volumes
Tx:	Oxybutynin Intermittent / Indwelling Catheter
F/u:	Too much antispasmodics → hypotonic

HYPOTONIC BLADDER / OVERFLOW INCONTINENCE	
Path:	Absent detrusor muscle contractions Neural Injury = Trauma, MS, etc. Leaks before ruptures
Pt:	⊘ Urge to void + Nocturnal Sxs Leak throughout day

Dx:	Physical = Normal . . . focal
	    neurologic deficit
	U/A = Normal
	Cystometry = no spasms at any
	    volume

Tx:	Bethanechol Intermittent / Indwelling Catheter

Adnexal Mass

DERMOID CYST / TERATOMA	
Path:	Benign tumor of ovary
Pt:	Young women (teens) Abdominal / Adnexal mass Weight Gain
Dx:	Ultrasound = Complex cyst
Tx:	Cystectomy (this cyst only)
F/u:	Likely to recur on the opposite side

ENDOMETRIOMA	
Path:	Retrograde Menses? Estrogen responsive tissues Endometrium outside the uterus
Pt:	Dysmenorrhea Dyspareunia Infertility
Dx:	U/S = Cyst Dx Lap with Laser Ablation OCP Trial
Tx:	1. Pelvic pain: NSAIDs 2. Axis: OCPs → GnRh analogues → Danazol 3. Dx Lap with Laser Ablation
F/u:	Chocolate cyst

ECTOPIC PREGNANCY	
Path:	Salpingitis (PID) = stricture Early fertilization Ampulla is most common site
Pt:	Amenorrhea / Spotting Abd Pain UPT +
Dx:	UPT + β-hCG (β-Quant) ≥ 2000 U/S = Ectopic

Tx:	Salpingostomy: no rupture
	Salpingectomy: + rupture
	MTX +/- Leucovorin
	  - β-hCG < 5000 (8,000)
	  - GS < 3 cm (3.5 cm)
	  - No heart tones

F/u:	Trend hCG to 0 . . . risk of Chorio

TUBO-OVARIAN ABSCESS	
Path:	PID = Gc / Chla Vaginal Flora

Pt:	Abd / Pelvic Pain
	No Other Cause
	1 of 3:
	  - Cervical Motion Tenderness
	  - Adnexal Tenderness
	  - Uterine Tenderness
	Fever, Leukocytosis
	+ WBC on wet prep ↑↑↑↑

Dx:	U/S = Abscess, Complex Cyst

Tx:	Inpatient IV
	  - Cefoxitin + Doxy + MTZ
	  - Clinda + Genta
	Drain
	  - If abx fail

F/u:	Drain if no improvement Cefoxitin + Doxycycline are for PID

TORSION OF THE OVARY	

Path:	Ovary twists about the vascular
	  supply and kills off the ovary
	Weight of the cysts, twists around the
	  suspensory ligament

Pt:	Spontaneous Abdominal Pain Toxic (Fever, Leuko) No good reason why
Dx:	U/S with Doppler = ↓ Flow

Tx:	Operate = Untwist
	  - Pinks up: leave it in
	  - Stays grey: cut it out

CYSTS	
Simple	Complex
Single, fluid filled, Homogeneous	Loculated, Lobulated, multiple Septations
Cystic	Solid, Mixed
Unilocular	Multilocular
< 7 cm	≥ 7 cm
Resolved in 2 months	Won't resolve
Treat with OCP	Already on OCP at diagnosis

CANCER
See the cancer section above

Pelvic Anatomy

POSTPARTUM HEMORRHAGE	
Path:	500cc Vaginal delivery
Pt:	1000cc C-section delivery

Tx:	1. NonSurgical
	    - Uterine Massage
	    - Medications
	        - Oxytocin
	        - Methergine
	        - Hemabate
	    - Balloon Tamponade
	
	2. Surgical
	    - Uterine Artery Ligation
	    - Internal Iliac Art Ligation
	    - Total Abdominal Hysterectomy

PELVIC FLOOR RELAXATION	
Path:	Multiple large births Stretched cardinal ligament
Pt:	Vaginal Fullness Chronic Back pain Speculum
Dx:	Clinical, physical exam

Tx:	1. Nonsurgical
	    Pessaries (conservative)
	
	2. Surgical
	    Hysterectomy (uterine)
	    Colporrhaphy (rectocele)
	    Colporrhaphy (cystocele)

F/u:	Dz-Specific
	    - Cystocele = Incontinence
	    - Rectocele = Constipation

CYSTOCELE	
Path:	Pelvic Floor relaxation
Pt:	Stress incontinence
Dx:	Clinical, physical exam - Cystocele falls down from the top
Tx:	Colporrhaphy (cystocele, rectocele)
F/u:	Stress incontinence

RECTOCELE	
Path:	Pelvic Floor relaxation
Pt:	Constipation
Dx:	Clinical, physical exam - Rectocele falls in from the bottom
Tx:	Colporrhaphy (cystocele, rectocele)
F/u:	Vaginal discharge

UTERINE PROLAPSE	
Path:	Pelvic Floor Relaxation
Pt:	Uterus visible in the vaginal canal, or outside the vagina Grade I: In vaginal canal Grade II: At vaginal opening Grade III: Out of vagina but not inverted Grade IV: inverted and out of the vagina
Dx:	Clinical
Tx:	Surgery

Gyn Infections

CANDIDAL VULVOVAGINITIS	
Path:	Disruption of the normal flora and pH
Pt:	Vaginal Discharge + Pruritus Sticky-White discharge Adherent to wall
Dx:	KOH prep = Hyphae Wet Prep = nothing pH > 4
Tx:	Fluconazole Topical → Po

BACTERIAL VAGINOSIS	
Path:	Gardnerella vaginalis
Pt:	Vaginal Discharge + Pruritus Whiff test Fishy odors Grey-white discharge
Dx:	Wet Prep = Clue Cells KOH prep = nothing pH > 5 (base)
Tx:	Metronidazole Topical → PO

TRICHOMONIASIS	
Path:	STD
Pt:	Vaginal Discharge + Pruritus Yellow-Green Discharge, Frothy Strawberry Cervix
Dx:	Wet Prep = Flagellated Motile organisms KOH prep = nothing pH > 5 (base)
Tx:	Metronidazole PO to BOTH PARTNERS

CERVICITIS	
Path:	Inflammation of Cervix Gc/Chla Vulvovaginitis
Pt:	+ Cervical Motion Tenderness + Cervical Discharge ∅ s/s of PID
Dx:	Physical Gc / Chla NAAT = PCR Wet Prep Gram Stain, Culture
Tx:	GC = Ceftriaxone IM x 1 Chla = Doxy x 7 or Azithro x 1

ACUTE PELVIC INFLAMMATORY DISEASE	
Path:	Ascending Infection GC 1/3 Chla 1/3 Vaginal Flora 1/3

Pt:	Abd / Pelvic Pain
	No Other Cause
	1 of 3:
	    - Cervical Motion Tenderness
	    - Adnexal Tenderness
	    - Uterine Tenderness
	Fever, Leukocytosis
	+ WBC on wet prep ↑↑↑

Dx:	Clx TV U/S = TOA, Free Fluid
Tx:	Inpt = Severe, N/V, Pregnant 1. Cefoxitin + Doxycycline 2. Clinda + Gentamycin Outpt = no need for inpt Ceftriaxone IM + Doxy + MTZ
F/u:	Surgery

TOXIC SHOCK SYNDROME	
Path:	S. aureus toxin, infection Toxin TSST-1 Tampons in too long

Pt:	Fever > 102
	Nausea / Vomiting and Diarrhea
	Erythematous, Macular,
	    Desquamating Rash of palms and
	    soles

Dx:	Other tests negative including blood cultures Speculum Exam
Tx:	Remove tampon Treat Staph: Nafcillin Treat Toxin: IVF (a lot), Support

Vaginal Bleeding: Premenarche

LIFE THREATENING BLEEDS	
Bleed	1. 2 Large Bore IV 2. IVF Bols 3. Type and Cross 4. IV Estrogen 5. Surgical Intervention
Surgery	- Intracavitary Tamponade - D&C - Uterine Art Embolization - Total Abdo Hysterectomy

BLEEDING BY AGE	
Premenarchal	Foreign Body Sexual Abuse Precocious Puberty Exam Under Anesthesia
Reproductive	Pregnancy Anatomy DUB = AUB Cervical Cancer UPT
Menopausal	Vaginal Atrophy Endometrial Cancer HRT Endometrial Biopsy

FOREIGN BODY	
Path:	Kids stick things in weird places
Pt:	Vaginal Bleeding without 2° sex char
Dx:	Exam under anesthesia
Tx:	Removal of object

SEXUAL ABUSE	
Path:	See peds, abuse
Pt:	Vaginal Bleeding without 2° sex char
Dx:	Exam under anesthesia
Tx:	Notify protective services, counseling

Vaginal Bleeding: Reproductive Years

ABORTION			
Diagnosis	Passage of Contents	Cervical OS	Ultrasound
IUP	None	Closed	Live Baby
Threatened	None	Closed	Live Baby
Inevitable	None	Open	Dead Baby
Incomplete	+	Open	Retained Parts
Complete	+	Closed	No Baby
---	---	---	---
Missed	None	Closed	Dead Baby

Do an ultrasound after the contents pass
Do track β-Quant to 0 to screen for trophoblastic disease
Do give IVIG to an Rh- mom at the time of abortion unless baby is absolutely known to be Rh-
Do induce a missed abortion (> 24 weeks)
Do remove a missed abortion (< 24 weeks)

ECTOPIC PREGNANCY	
Path:	Zygote implants not in uterus MC = Ampulla Stricture
Pt:	Abdominal Pain, Bleeding UPT +
Dx:	B-Quant and TV ultrasound

Tx:	Salpingostomy: ∅ rupture
	Salpingectomy: + rupture
	Methotrexate ok if
	  - GC < 3 cm (3.5)
	  - β-hCG < 5000 (8000)
	  - No heart tones

F/u:	β-Quant
	  - If < 1500, check in 48 hrs
	  - If < 2000, look at ultrasound
	  - If β-hCG doubles = IUP

Vaginal Bleeding: Anatomy

FIBROIDS	
Path:	Benign Estrogen-Responsive myometrium
Pt:	Asymmetric, Nodular uterus Bleeding / Anemia Infertility Painful Visceral Obstruction
Dx:	1st = Ultrasound Best = MRI

Tx:	Meds
	  - NSAID
	  - OCPs
	Surgery
	  - Wants kids → Myomectomy
	  - ∅ Want kids → TAH
	  - Too Big → GnRH Analogs
	    (Leuprolide)

POLYCYSTIC OVARIAN SYNDROME	
Path:	Anovulation → Estrogen ∅ Progesterone Atretic Follicles → Testosterone
Pt:	Hirsute = Fat + Hairy Deep Voice Anemia Infertility Endometrial Cancer

Dx:	~~Ultrasound → 1000s of follicles~~ (not
	  needed)
	LH/FSH > 3
	Endocrine: ↑ T, Normal DHEAS
	Diabetes—2-hour glucose test OR
	  A1c

Tx:	OCPs Metformin Clomiphene

DYSFUNCTIONAL UTERINE BLEEDING	

Path:	Atretic Follicles
	No Ovulation = No progesterone =
	  Estrogen only = Proliferation
	NORMAL near menarche near
	  menopause

Pt:	Bleeding that occurs without regular cycles

Dx:	Diagnosis of exclusion. Rule out
	  everything else with . . .
	CBC, TSH, U/S, MRI, Prolactin,
	  Hysteroscopy, etc.

Tx:	~~↓ Stress~~ ~~↑ Weight~~ OCPs—anemia NSAIDs
F/u:	Very significant bleeding = IV estrogen Unresponsive to IV estrogen, TAH

GYN

Vaginal Bleeding: Puberty

PRECOCIOUS PUBERTY	

Path:	Estrogen
	  - Estrogen should come from
	    ovaries
	  - Estrogen drives the uterus to
	    bleed
	HPA Axis
	Hypothalamus
	Anterior Pituitary = LH/FSH
	  secreting tumor
	Ovarian Cyst = Cyst, Granulosa-
	  Theca tumor
	Adrenal Tumor = CAH and Adrenal
	  Tumor

Pt:	Early < 8 year old 2° sex characteristics

Dx:	Wrist X-ray Bone Age. Bone Age
	  > 2 years chronological age =
	  precocious puberty
	GnRH Stim Test
	= Central Precocious Puberty if LH ↑
	  - MRI separates tumor from
	    constitutional
	= Peripheral Precocious Puberty if
	  LH ∅ Δ
	  - U/S separates ovarian from
	    adrenal

Tx:	Constitutional: Leuprolide Tumor: Resection CAH: Steroids (see Virilization) Cyst: Observe (simple), Resect (complex)

DELAYED PUBERTY	
Path:	See peds, Abuse
Pt:	∅ 2° sex char by 13 ∅ Bleeding by 15

Dx:	Bone Age, FSH, LH
	  - ↑ FSH, ↑ LH = Karyotype
	  - ∅ FSH, ∅LH = find disease

Tx:	If there is a disease, treat
F/u:	Constitutional delay if family history, just wait NEVER GH

Primary Amenorrhea

PRIMARY AMENORRHEA	
Path:	Axis—intact HPA axis → Breasts Anatomy—uterus → Uterus
Pt:	No 2° sex char by 13 No menarche by 15
Dx:	Urine Pregnancy Test Wrist X-ray Ultrasound of the Uterus
Tx:	Disease specific

CONSTITUTIONAL AND COMMON CAUSES	
Path:	Hypothalamus controls everything
Pt:	Anorexia Weight loss, Intense exercise Pregnancy before the first period
Dx:	1st: Urinary Pregnancy Test Clinical
Tx:	Reassurance Ultrasound only if pregnant

CRANIOPHARYNGIOMA + KALLMANN	
Path:	Hypothalamus
Pt:	+ Uterus ∅ Breast Development No menarche
Dx:	FSH / LH ↓ MRI (∅ Mass Kallmann, + mass Cranio)
Tx:	Estrogen + Progesterone Resection
F/u:	Kallmann has anosmia

MULLERIAN AGENESIS	
Path:	Genetically Female (X,X) Idiopathic Loss of mullerian ducts
Pt:	+ 2° Sex + ♀ External Genitalia ∅ Uterus, ∅ Tubes, ∅ no upper 1/3rd vagina
Dx:	1st: Ultrasound = No uterus Karyotype = (X,X) FSH/LH normal
Tx:	Elevate Vagina Adopt, cannot get pregnant

CAUSES BASED ON THE METHOD		
Axis	Anatomy	
+	+	Pregnancy, Anorexia, Weight loss, Imperforate Hymen
+	-	Mullerian Agenesis, Testicular Feminization
-	+	Craniopharyngioma, Kallmann syndrome, Turner's
-	-	Beyond the scope of this course; don't worry about it.

TURNER SYNDROME	
Path:	Streak Ovaries Genetically (X,O)
Pt:	Web Neck Broad spaced nipples Cardiac Issues
Dx:	1st: Ultrasound = Positive uterus, streak ovaries Karyotype = (X,O) . . . (X,X) FSH/LH ↑
Tx:	Estrogen and Progesterone
F/u:	Echocardiogram—coarctation

ANDROGEN INSENSITIVITY SYNDROME	
Path:	Genetically Male (X,Y) Has testes but looks female on the outside Resistant to Testosterone
Pt:	+ 2° Sex + ♀ External Genitalia ∅ Uterus
Dx:	1st: Ultrasound = No uterus Karyotype = (X,Y) FSH/LH normal
Tx:	Elevate Vagina Remove testicles after puberty
F/u:	Formerly known as Testicular Feminization

GYN

Secondary Amenorrhea

COMMON CAUSES	
Pregnancy	Urinary Pregnancy Test
Hypothyroid	TSH
Prolactin	Prolactin
- emia	
- oma	
Medications	Dopamine Antagonist
HPA Axis	The rest of the section

HYPOTHYROIDISM	
Path:	↑ TRH stimulates Ant Pit to produce Prolactin → prolactinemia
Pt:	Hypothyroidism (endocrine)
Dx:	TSH, T4 ~~Prolactin level~~
Tx:	Levothyroxine

ANTI-PSYCHOTICS	
Path:	Dopamine-Antagonists disinhibit Prolactin → Prolactinemia
Pt:	Schizophrenia, Mood disorders Antipsychotics
Dx:	~~Prolactin level~~
Tx:	Tolerate the side effects, change drugs

PREGNANCY	
Path:	Check a UPT with any amenorrhea

HYPOTHALAMIC CAUSES	
Path:	Hypothalamus controls everything
Pt:	Anorexia, Weight loss, extreme exercise
Dx:	Clinical UPT
Tx:	Supportive

PROLACTINOMA	
Path:	Pituitary Adenoma
Pt:	Galactorrhea and Amenorrhea
Dx:	UPT and TSH Prolactin MRI
Tx:	Dopamine-Agonists (pramipexole, ropinerole, bromocriptine)
	Surgery if refractory

SAVAGE SYNDROME (THE OTHER MENOPAUSE)	
Path:	Unresponsive Ovaries
Pt:	Young woman going through menopause who shouldn't
Dx:	Progestin negative E+P Challenge induces bleed FSH,LH ↑↑ Ultrasound + Follicles
Tx:	Supportive

MENOPAUSE	
Path:	Unresponsive Ovaries
Pt:	50ish year old woman going through menopause who should be
Dx:	Clinical ~~Progestin negative~~ ~~E+P Challenge induces bleed~~ ~~FSH,LH ↑↑~~ ~~Ultrasound + Follicles~~
Tx:	Supportive
F/u:	venlafaxine for hot flashes

ABLATION	
Path:	We caused burns to the endometrium
Pt:	s/p ablation
Dx:	Clinical
Tx:	None

ASHERMAN'S SYNDROME	
Path:	Frequent surgeries, elective abortions, scarring
Pt:	Frequent procedures
Dx:	Fails progestin challenge (can't bleed)
Tx:	None

Infertility

ERECTILE DYSFUNCTION	
Path:	♂ fault
Pt:	Psychogenic or Organic
Dx:	Night-Time Tumescence
Tx:	Psychogenic: Counseling Organic: Sildenafil
F/u:	Always blame the dude first

IDIOPATHIC
All other tests have failed to find a cause
Adoption
Surrogate, ICSI

INHOSPITABLE MUCOUS	
Path:	Soft mucous needed
Pt:	Inability to conceive
Dx:	Mucous Workup - Smush test < 6 cm smush - No sperm - No fern sign
Tx:	Estrogen Bypass = Artificial Insemination

OVULATION ISSUES	
Path:	♀ fault
Pt:	Inability to conceive Normal mucous workup

Dx:	Basal Temp rises 1° on ovulation
	Endometrial biopsy day 14-28 =
	    secretory uterus
	Progesterone levels at day 22
	Hx . . . anovulatory = h/o irregular
	    menses

Tx:	Clomiphene Pergonal

ANATOMIC ISSUES	
Path:	♀ fault Fibroids (implantation), Stricture, PID (tubes)
Pt:	Inability to conceive Normal mucous, normal ovulation
Dx:	Hysterosalpingogram
Tx:	ICSI, in vitro fertilization, Surrogate Tuboplasty

ENDOMETRIOSIS	
Path:	♀ fault Retrograde Flow
Pt:	Abdominal pain, dyspareunia
Dx:	Ex-Lap with Laser Ablation
Tx:	Laser Ablation

Menopause

MENOPAUSE	
Path:	Ovarian failure - Estrogen ↓
Pt:	Hot Flashes Vaginal Atrophy ↓ Libido Irritability / Mood Swings Cessation of menstrual periods for 12 cycles
Dx:	Clinical ↑ FSH ↑ LH ↓ Estrogen
Tx:	Phytoestrogen Hormone replacement therapy Venlafaxine Vaginal creams
F/u:	Osteoporosis → give Ca + Vit D Dexa scan at 65 CAD → Lipid Panel → Statin

Virilization

DEFINITIONS	
Hirsute:	Weight Gain and Hair Growth Small amount of androgen
Virilized:	Weight and Hair growth plus Clitoromegaly, Deep Voice, Muscles Severe amount of androgen
Ovaries:	Testosterone
Adrenals:	DHEAS
Cancers:	Severe elevations, unilateral
Noncancer:	Mild elevations, bilateral

POLYCYSTIC OVARIAN DISEASE	
Path:	Noncancer problem of the ovaries resulting from anovulation. Atretic follicles produce testosterone
Pt:	Hirsute, trouble getting pregnant
Dx:	Testosterone ↑ DHEAS normal Ultrasound = Bilateral Ovarian Follicles LH/FHS ratio 3:1
Tx:	Metformin (insulin insensitivity) Oral Contraception (atretic follicles) Spironolactone (hair growth) Clomiphene for pregnancy
F/u:	Endocrine diagnosis, you do not need to have the ultrasound to make the diagnosis.

SERTOLI-LEYDIG TUMOR	
Path:	Cancer of the ovary that autonomously secretes Testosterone
Pt:	Virilization
Dx:	Ultrasound = Unilateral Mass - Testosterone ↑↑↑ - DHEAS normal
Tx:	Resection (usually benign)

ADRENAL TUMOR	
Path:	Cancer of the adrenal gland that autonomously secretes DHEAS
Pt:	Virilization
Dx:	Ultrasound = Unilateral Mass - Testosterone Normal - DHEAS ↑↑↑ Bilateral Adrenal Vein sampling
Tx:	Resection (usually benign)

CONGENITAL ADRENAL HYPERPLASIA	
Path:	21-α-hydroxylase deficiency or inability to make cortisol and aldosterone such that there is too much DHEAS instead
Pt:	Either Virilization or Hirsute
Dx:	Ultrasound = Bilateral adrenals - DHEAS ↑ - Testosterone Normal *** Urinary 17-OH-Progesterone ***
Tx:	Cortisol Fludrocortisone

FAMILIAL HIRSUTISM	
Path:	Genetic trait that makes people hairy
Pt:	Hirsutism
Dx:	Normal Diagnostics Ultrasound Normal - DHEAS Normal - Testosterone Normal - FSH/LH Normal
Tx:	None needed, cosmetic

Physiology of Pregnancy

CARDIOVASCULAR CHANGES	
↓ SVR	↓ BP
↑ CO	↑ Preload, ↑ HR, Normal EF
↑ RBC	↑ Oxygen Delivery
↑↑ Plasma	↓ Hgb (despite more RBCs)

COAGULATION	
↑ vWF	↑ Primary hemostasis
↑ VII, VIII, X	↑ Secondary hemostasis
↓ C, S	↑ Secondary hemostasis
↑ Fibrinogen (I)	Normal levels indicate pathology
↑ D-Dimer	Useless test in pregnancy

PULMONARY	
FEV1	No change
PaO$_2$	No Change
Functional residual capacity	↓
Minute Ventilation	Tv ↑, RR no change

GU	
↑ GFR	↓ Cr
Obstructive Uropathy	Ureters pelvic brim

WEIGHT GAIN		
BMI	Total Weight	Rate of Gain
< 18.5	28-40 lbs	1 lb / week
18.5-24.9	25-35 lbs	0.75 lb / week
25-29.9	15-25 lbs	0.5 lb / week
> 30	11-20 lbs	0.25 /lb / week

GASTROINTESTINAL	
GERD	PPI
Constipation Nausea Iron supplements Gallstones	Stool softener, motility Ondansetron PPx constipation

ENDOCRINE	
Estrogen	Hypercoagulable
Prolactin	Nipple discharge

Normal Prenatal Care

WHAT TO EVALUATE	
Safety and Risk	Genetic disease Carrier states Domestic violence Maternal complications
Folic Acid	Neural Tube Defects
Vaccinations	Influenza Hep B MMR (live attenuated)
Lifestyle	Smoking cessation Alcohol cessation Exercise Sleep Stress management
Optimize pre-existing disease	Diabetes Hypertension Thyroid

FIRST VISIT	
Timing	10 weeks gestational age
Testing	Urine screen U/S confirms β-hCG serum rarely needed
The Person	Desire for pregnancy, counseling Barriers to care Screen for violence at home Vitals, Weight, Height
The Pregnancy	GPA or TPAL Zika and Ebola exposure
Follow-up	q4w until 28, q2w until 36, q1w

FIRST TRIMESTER LABS	
Blood	
ABO type Rh Ag	Alloimmunization risk ("Rh status")
Hgb/Hct	Baseline Hgb Identify correctable anemia
Rubella	Assess immunity (cannot give MMRV)
Varicella	Assess immunity (cannot give MMRV)
HIV	Confirm and viral load if positive
RPR	Syphilis screen
Hep B	Antigen status Antibody status
Cytology	
Pap	Pap if indicated by age and history (This might be the time to capture her)
Urine	

U/A,
  Ucx
	Screen for and treat asymptomatic
	  bacteriuria

Protein	Confounds eclampsia picture
GC/Chla	Treat both if you find one

Genetic Diseases

ANEUPLOIDY		
Disease	*Memory Tool*	*Chromosome*
Down's	Drinking Age	21
Edwards	Election Age	18
Patau	The other one (also PG-13 movies)	13

SCREENING AND DIAGNOSTIC TESTING	
Screening	Identifies Risk, not diagnosis
If High Risk	Invasive Procedure
If Low Risk	Reassurance

RISK OF ANEUPLOIDY	
↑ maternal age - Fewer pregnancies - Higher risk	RISK is high
Normal maternal age - Many pregnancies - Lower risk	PREVALENCE is high

FIRST TRIMESTER MARKERS			
	PAPP-A	hCG	NT
Down's	↓	↑	↑
18	↓↓	↓↓	↑
13	↓↓	↓	↑

SECOND TRIMESTER MARKERS			
	Tri Screen		Quad
	hCG	AFP	Estriol	InhibinA
Down's	↑	↓	↓	↑
18	↓↓	↓	↓↓	-
13	-	-	-	-

Third Trimester Labs

GESTATIONAL DIABETES (NOT CHRONIC DIABETES)	
Path:	Insulin insensitivity Preconception Obesity 1lb / week gain Advanced maternal age
Pt:	Asx Screen

Dx:	1 hr glucose tolerance test 50g: + > 140
	3 hr glucose tolerance test 100g:
	  - Fasting ≥ 95
	  - 1 hr ≥ 180
	  - 2 hr ≥ 155
	  - 3 hr ≥ 140
	  - Positive if 2 of 4
	~~Hgb A1c~~
	~~Fasting Glucose~~

Tx:	Insulin → qHs qAc ~~Oral~~
F/u:	Oral agents (Metformin and Glyburide are ok if a patient won't take insulin. Insulin is still the right answer)

ANEMIA	
Path:	Hemoglobin Nadir 28-36 weeks Iron deficiency
Pt:	Asx Screen
Dx:	CBC—Anemia only if < 10 / < 30 ↓ MCV ↓ Ferritin ~~Bone Marrow Biopsy~~
Tx:	Iron
F/u:	Prophylaxis with Folate is not for anemia, but for baby's development.

ISOIMMUNIZATION (FULL LECTURE LATER)	

Path:	Rh- Mom and Rh+ Dad = Rh+ Baby
	Rh- Mom and Rh+ Baby =
	  Rh-IgM → Rh-IgG
	Rh- Mom and Rh+ Baby and Rh-IgG
	  = Anemia
	Isoimmunization during delivery/ procedure

Pt:	Asx screen
	  - Rh status at first visit
	  - Rh antibody status at 24 weeks

Dx:	Mom's Rh status (must be Rh- to matter) Dad Rh+ or Unknown Get Rh antibody for mom
Tx:	Rh- Mom and Rh-Ab-Neg = Rhogam at 28 weeks and 72 hours from delivery Rh- mom and Rh-Ab-Pos = Too Late

Advanced Prenatal Evaluation

Procedure	Gestational Age	Goal	Risk of Loss	Bonus
Ultrasound	Any	Intrauterine Pregnancy Fetal age Fetal Well-being	No risk	1st Trimester +/- 1 week 2nd Trimester +/- 2 weeks 3rd Trimester +/- 3 weeks
Transcranial Doppler	> 20 weeks	Screen for fetal anemia (Alloimmunization)	No risk	No access (compare to PUBS)
Amniocentesis	> 16 weeks	AFP, Genetics, fetal lung maturity, assess for infection	0.1-0.3%	> 16 weeks: Genetic > 24 weeks: Liley Graph > 36 weeks: L:S ratio
Chorionic Villous Sampling	10-12 weeks	Genetics, Karyotyping	0.22%	None
Percutaneous Umbilical Cord Sampling	> 20 weeks AND < 32 weeks	Confirm Fetal Anemia Treat Fetal Anemia		Access for transfusion Just deliver if > 32 weeks

Listed in order of ascending risk of fetal demise.

Medical Disease

ASX BACTERIURIA	
Path:	Gram Negatives, Group B Strep
Pt:	Asx Screen, NO symptoms
Dx:	U/A positive
Tx:	Amoxicillin (1st line) Nitrofurantoin (if pen allergic) *TMP-SMX* ~~Cipro~~
F/u:	DO rescreen a pregnant woman (normally you don't)

CYSTITIS (UTI)	
Path:	Gram Negatives, Group B Strep
Pt:	Urgency, Frequency, Dysuria
Dx:	U/A positive
Tx:	Amoxicillin (1st line) Nitrofurantoin (if pen allergic) *TMP-SMX* ~~Cipro~~
F/u:	DO rescreen a pregnant woman (normally you don't) Treat for 7 days (complicated UTI)

PYELONEPHRITIS	
Path:	Gram Negatives, Group B Strep
Pt:	Urgency, Frequency, Dysuria Fevers, Chills, Nausea, Vomiting CVA Tenderness
Dx:	U/A positive, WBC casts
Tx:	Ceftriaxone
F/u:	If no improvement after 3 days, Ultrasound looking for abscess. ~~CT scan abdomen~~

HYPERTENSION	
Path:	Goal < 140 / < 90 Onset before 20 weeks gestation
Pt:	ASX Screen, Vitals every visit
Dx:	Ambulatory BP
Tx:	α-methyl-dopa best answer Labetalol Hydralazine ~~ACE-inhibitors, ARBs, Thiazide~~
F/u:	Strict screening for Eclampsia

THYROID	
Path:	Hyperthyroid—dead baby Hypothyroid—Cretinism, MR
Pt:	Hyper: ↑ Hypo: ↓
Dx:	Hyper: ↓ TSH with ↑ T4 ... ~~RAIU~~ Hypo: ↑ TSH with ↓ T4
Tx:	Hyper: PTU is safe in Pregnancy If surgery, do it 2nd trimester ~~Radioactive I Ablation~~ Hypo: Levothyroxine
F/u:	↑ Thyroid Binding Globulin means ↑ Levothyroxine ~25% Trend TSH q4weeks (not q12weeks)

SEIZURE	
Path:	"All Antiepileptics are teratogens"
Pt:	Epilepsy
Dx:	Clinical
Tx:	Risk benefit analysis ↑ Frequency = ↑ Treatment ↑ Severity (grand mal) = ↑ Treatment If able, Avoid during 1st trimester Levetiracetam or Lamotrigine OK ~~Valproate, Valproic Acid~~ (X) ~~Phenytoin~~ (D) ~~Carbamazepine~~ (D)
F/u:	Phenobarbital for Pregnancy to abort seizures (benzos ok, especially if late in pregnancy) Folate for all women on AED looking to get pregnant

DIABETES (NOT GESTATIONAL)	
Path:	Type I: Autoimmune Destruction Pancreas Type II: Obesity, Insulin Sensitivity
Pt:	↑ bG, fasting glucose, or A1c
Dx:	A1c
Tx:	Pre-Pregnancy Weight loss, diet, exercise Oral medications → Insulin Maximize regimen, A1c < 7 During Pregnancy ↑ Insulin requirements Basal Bolus A1c is useless! Post = Pregnancy ↓ Insulin demands at delivery (rapid) Macrosomia, Shoulder dystocia (Tri 3) Transposition of great vessels (Tri 1)

Normal Labor

STAGES OF LABOR	
Stage I	Latent Phase: Onset of contractions 0 cm → 6 cm - 20 hrs (nulli) - 14 hrs (multi) Active Phase: 6 cm → 10 cm - 1.2 cm / hr (nulli) - 1.5 cm / hr (multi) - 5 hrs max
Stage II	10 cm → baby delivered - 3 hrs (nulli) - 2 hrs (multi) - + 1 hr for epidural
Stage III	Baby delivered → Placenta delivered
Stage IV	Done

CERVICAL CHANGES	
Changes	Softening (literally softer) Dilation (opening) Effacement (shortening) Position (aims baby for ejection)
Path:	Breakage of Disulfide Bonds Collagen breaks, water fills
Tx:	Fetal head stimulates change Balloon simulates fetal head PGE2, Amniotomy

FETAL STATION	
-5	# of centimeters from 0, away from vaginal opening
0	Ischial Spines
+5	# of centimeters from 0, towards vaginal opening

ABNORMAL FETAL POSITION ("BREECH")	
Path:	Leopold maneuver @ wk 37
Dx:	Ultrasound
Tx:	External Version C-section

FETAL POSITIONS	
Longitudinal	Baby and mom parallel
Transverse	Baby and mom perpendicular
Longitudinal Cephalic	The only normal presentation; baby head down
Footling Breech	Hips EXTENDED knees don't matter
Complete Breech	Hips FLEXED Knees flexed
Frank Breech	Hips FLEXED Knees extended

Abnormal Labor

PROLONGED LATENT PHASE	
Path:	Inadequate contractions Contractions to 6 cm dilation
Pt:	20 hrs (nulli) 14 hrs (multi)
Tx:	Balloon to stimulate engagement Misoprostol Oxytocin Amniotomy

PROLONGED ACTIVE PHASE	
Path:	Power, Passenger, Pelvis 6 cm to 10 cm

Pt:	Prolonged active phase
	  - 1.5 cm / hr (nulli)
	  - 1.2 cm / hr (multi)
	Arrest of active phase
	  - 4 hrs adequate ctx
	  - 6 hrs all comer

Tx:	Frequency / Adequacy: Oxytocin Everything else: C-section

PROLONGED 2ND STAGE	
Path:	Power, Passenger, Pelvis 10 cm to Baby delivered
Pt:	3 hrs (nulli) 2 hrs (multi)
Tx:	Negative station: C-section Positive station: Vaginal operations Forceps = Vacuum

PROLONGED 3RD STAGE	
Path:	Power only Baby delivered to Placenta Delivered
Pt:	30 minutes
Tx:	Uterine Massage Oxytocin Manual Extraction

CONTRACTIONS	
Adequacy	> 200 Montevideo units in 10 mins
Method	Intrauterine pressure catheter
Frequency	3 ctx in 10 minutes

L & D Pathology

RUPTURE OF MEMBRANES	

Path:	Term baby (baby is ready)
	Contractions (mom is ready)
	Normal process of delivery
	  - Spontaneous (mom's ready)
	  - Artificially (to help mom
	    progress)

Pt:	Rush of fluid—meconium, blood, clear
Dx:	Speculum exam shows pooling of fluid Nitrazine test turns blue Ferning on a glass slide
Tx:	Deliver

pROM (PREMATURE RUPTURE OF MEMBRANES)	
Path:	Term baby (baby is ready) Absent Contractions (Mom is not)
Pt:	ROM but no contractions
Dx:	Same as ROM Check GBS status
Tx:	Induce labor +/- GBS abx

ppROM (PRETERM PREMATURE RUPTURE OF MEM)	
Path:	Preterm baby (baby not ready) No contractions (mom not ready) ROM happens anyway
Pt:	Rush of fluid—meconium, blood, clear
Dx:	Same as ROM
Tx:	> 34 weeks—deliver 24-34 wks—corticosteroids < 24 weeks—nonviable
F/u:	Abx

PROLONGED ROM	
Path:	Term baby (baby is ready) Contractions (mom is ready) GBS is the real risk
Pt:	ROM . . . AND . . . > 18 hours
Dx:	Clinical
Tx:	GBS + or Unknown: Abx GBS - : watch and wait
F/u:	Chorioamnionitis and Endometritis

CHORIOAMNIONITIS / ENDOMETRITIS	
Path:	Ascending infection from vagina Chorio: Baby still in mom Endom: Baby out of mom
Pt:	Fever, sepsis, toxic If prolonged ROM, ↑ risk
Dx:	Rule out others: X-ray, U/A, Blood Vaginal culture (contaminated)
Tx:	Amp + Gent + Clinda Cipro + Metronidazole

PRETERM LABOR	
Path:	Leading cause of morbidity and mortality for neonates
Pt:	Contractions with Cervical Δ Gestational age 21-36 weeks
Dx:	Clinical
Tx:	< 34 weeks: STEROIDS and tocolytics < 20 weeks: nonviable
F/u:	Lecithin/Sphingomyelin ratio Amniocentesis Tocolytics are really to get mom to a tertiary center

POST DATES	
Path:	-----
Pt:	Baby > 40 weeks by conception Baby > 42 weeks by menstrual cycle
Dx:	Certainty of gestational age?
Tx:	> 42 weeks—induce, C/S if failed induction
F/u:	Macrosomic, Shoulder Dystocia, meconium aspiration, fetal demise

Eclampsia

	BLOOD PRESSURE	TIMING	URINE	SYMPTOMS	TREATMENT
Transient HTN (tHTN)	≥ 140 / ≥ 90	**Unsustained** any time	∅	∅	**Conservative Keep a Log**
Chronic HTN (cHTN)	≥ 140 / ≥ 90	Sustained, Starting **before 20 weeks**	∅	∅	**α-methyldopa** Hydralazine Labetalol
Gestational HTN (gHTN)	≥ 140 / ≥ 90	Sustained, Starting **after 20 weeks**	∅	∅	**Monitor** for PEC
PreEclampsia without severe features (PEC)	**≥ 140 / ≥ 90**	Sustained, Starting **after 20 weeks**	**300mg/dL** proteinuria	∅	> 37 weeks **deliver** urgently (induced) < 37 weeks **bed rest**
PreEclampsia with severe features (sPEC)	**> 160 / > 110**	Sustained, Starting **after 20 weeks**	+/- **proteinuria**	Positive*	**Mag + BP** + deliver urgently (Induced)
Eclampsia	----	-----	----	**Seizures**	**Mag + Deliver** emergently (Section)
HELLP	Hemolysis	Elevated LFTs	Low	Platelets	**Mag + Deliver** emergently (Section)

SEVERE FEATURES = ALARM SXS		RISK BENEFIT OF NOT DELIVERING	
↓ Platelets	↑ Cr > 1.1 (2x	*RISK*	*BENEFIT*
↑ LFTs	baseline)	*Mortality*	*Fetal Development*
RUQ Abd Pain	Pulm Edema	*# of severe features*	*> 37 weeks: none*
	HA, Vision Changes	*severity of severe*	*24-37: decremental*
BP ≥ 160 / ≥ 110		*stability of mom*	*< 24 weeks: none*
		stability of baby	

Multiple Gestations

DI-ZYGOTIC DI-AMNIOTIC DI-CHORIONIC	
Path:	Two Eggs, Two Sperm Ø Split
Pt:	Babies are non-identical
Dx:	Ultrasound = Different Genders Two placentas Two sacs Two Fetuses
Risk:	IUGR Premature delivery (2-3 weeks / twin) Preeclampsia (3x) PPH Placental abruption Congenital anomalies
F/u:	can be same gender

MONO-ZYGOTIC DI-CHORIONIC DI-AMNIOTIC	
Path:	One egg Split 0-3 days (Tubal)
Pt:	Babies identical (same gender)
Dx:	Ultrasound = Same Genders Two placentas Two sacs Two Fetuses
Risk:	Same as above

MONO-ZYGOTIC MONO-CHORIONIC DI-AMNIOTIC	
Path:	One egg Split 4-8 days (Blastocyst)
Pt:	Babies identical (same gender)
Dx:	Ultrasound = Same Genders One placenta Two sacs Two Fetuses
Risk:	Same as above AND Twin-Twin Transfusion The transfusing twin does better

MONO-ZYGOTIC MONO-CHORIONIC MONO-AMNIOTIC	
Path:	One Egg Split - Day 9-12 (un-conjoined) - Day ≥ 12 (conjoined)
Pt:	Babies are identical
Dx:	Ultrasound = Same Genders One placenta One sac Two fetuses (conjoined or not)
Risk:	Same as above AND Cord Entanglement Conjoined Twins

OB

Post-Partum Hemorrhage

UTERINE ATONY	
Path:	Cannot contract down - Prolonged Labor - Oxytocin stopped - Tocolytics
Pt:	PPH + Boggy Uterus
Dx:	Clx
Tx:	Uterine Massage Methylergonovine Oxytocin PGF-2-α Surgery

DISSEMINATED INTRAVASCULAR COAGULATION		
Path:	Placental Contents Fibrin Clots Consume Plts, Factors	
Pt:	PPH Won't stop Oozing IV Sites	
Dx:	Plts ↓	Platelets
	Factors ↓	FFP
	Fibrinogen ↓	Cryo
	Smear ↓	pRBC

UTERINE INVERSION	
Path:	Uterus "births" itself - Oxytocin use - Umbilical traction
Pt:	PPH + Absent Uterus
Dx:	Clinical . . . Speculum
Tx:	Manual replacement - Tocolytics to ease placement - Oxytocin to contract down

VAGINAL LACERATIONS	
Path:	Precipitous Birth Macrosomic Babies Episiotomy
Pt:	PPH + Normal Uterus
Dx:	Clinical . . . Speculum
Tx:	Manual Pressure . . . sutures

RETAINED PLACENTA	
Path:	Placenta burrows deeply Accessory Lobe Placenta Tears Depth = Name
Pt:	PPH + Firm
Dx:	Clinical . . . Placenta blood vessel to edge
Tx:	1st D&C TAH
F/u:	β-hCG

Antenatal Testing

NON-STRESS TEST

Path:	Accelerations Variability
Good:	15, 15, 2 in 20—increase in the heart rate 15 bpm, 15 seconds occurring twice in 20 minutes
Bad:	Not 15, 15, 2 in 20 Do Vibroacoustic Stimulation

VIBROACOUSTIC STIMULATION TEST

Path:	Non-Stress Test But with vibroacoustic stim
Good:	15, 15, 2 in 20—increase in the heart rate 15 bpm, 15 seconds occurring twice in 20 minutes
Bad:	Not 15, 15, 2 in 20 Biophysical Profile

BIOPHYSICAL PROFILE

Path:	Ultrasound 0-2: Amniotic Fluid Index 0-2: NST 0-2: Breathing 0-2: Movement 0-2: Tone
Good:	8-10, repeat weekly
Bad:	0-2, deliver
Middle:	2-8, gestational age - > 36 weeks = deliver - < 36 Weeks = CST

CST AND DECELERATIONS

Early Decels:	Head Compressions, Nonworrisome
Variable Decels:	Cord Compressions, Nonworrisome
Late Decels:	Uteroplacental Insufficiency, Immediate Delivery

VEAL CHOP

Variable Decels	–	**C**ord Compression
Early Decels	–	**H**ead Compression
Accelerations	–	**O**kay
Late Decels	–	**P**lacental Insufficiency

Third Trimester Bleeding

PLACENTA PREVIA

Path:	Placenta implants across os Os dilates = Tears placenta Baby's Blood Risk: Multiple Gestations, Multiparous
Pt:	Pain<u>LESS</u> third tri bleed Baby doing poorly
Dx:	U/S= Transverse Lie C/NST = Fetal Distress
Tx:	C/S
F/u:	- Marginal: barely into os - Partial: halfway into os - Complete: across the os

PLACENTAL ABRUPTION

Path:	Tearing of the Placenta off mom HTN, Cocaine, MVA Mom's Blood
Pt:	PainFUL third trimester bleed Sudden Onset Pain
Dx:	U/S → Tear C/NST = Fetal Distress
Tx:	C/S
F/u:	Concealed Abruption

UTERINE RUPTURE

Path:	C/S Scar, ↑↑ VBAC Oxytocin Tears uterus apart . . . baby takes path of least resistance→birthed into peritoneum
Pt:	Pain<u>FUL</u> ± bleed Delivery . . . ↓ CTX, ↓ Fetal Heart Rate
Dx:	DON'T WAIT
Tx:	Crash Section

VASA PREVIA

Path:	Accessory lobe Blood vessels cross the os Os dilates = Blood Vessels Tear Baby's Blood
Pt:	Pain<u>LESS</u> 3rd trimester bleeding Fetal Distress
Dx:	~~U/S~~ C/NST → Fetal Distress
Tx:	C-Section

Alloimmunization

	ALLOIMMUNIZATION
Path:	**Genetics:** Mom is Rh-Ag-NEG + Dad is Rh-Ag-POS Therefore Baby is Rh-Ag-POS **Exposure** 1st Exposure (Baby 1) IgM, cannot cross placenta, when blood mixes = D&C, Delivery, Bleed Rh-Ab-Neg Mom → Rh-Ab-Pos Mom Rh-An-Neg Mom ??? Rh-Ag-Pos baby 2nd Exposure (Baby 2) IgG, can cross placenta, causes fetal anemia Rh-Ab-POS Mom ATTACKS Rh-Ag-Pos **Subtypes** **D**uffy **D**ies = anemia **K**al **K**ills = anemia **L**ewis **L**ives = no anemia Titers > 1:8

Dxs:	1st: Type and Screen, Mom's Rh-Ag-Status
	2nd: Dad's Ag status
	  - Type and Screen
	  - Amniocentesis PCR for baby's genotype
	3rd: Transcranial Doppler
	  - Decide treatment here on age
	
	Wrong Tests
	  ~~Liley Graph~~ (always wrong)
	  ~~PUBS~~ (you PUBS only to treat)

Tx:	GA < 32 weeks PUBS for transfusion GA ≥ 32 weeks Deliver
PPx:	Rho(D) Immune globulin for an Antibody Negative, Antigen Negative mom at 27 weeks and within 72 hours of delivery

Prenatal Infections

HEPATITIS B	
Path:	Hep B Vertical transmission Chronic carrier if vertical infection
Pt:	Mom has Hep B, high incidence in Asia Baby asx until Cirrhosis or HCC
Dx:	Mom Hep B s Ab = Immune Mom Hep B s Ag = infected Mom Hep B c Ab = Exposed Immune
Tx:	Vaccinate mom Get Hep B vaccine + Hep V IVIg

HERPES SIMPLEX VIRUS	
Path:	Hide in the dorsal root ganglion, then descend to the skin
Pt:	Painful prodrome Vesicles on an erythematous base
Dx:	Clinical, can do HSV PCR
Tx:	Acyclovir to mom, C-section to avoid lesion
F/u:	Viremia messes up baby, happens only on initial exposure.

SYPHILIS	
Path:	Treponema
Pt:	Painless ulcer Targetoid lesion on palms and soles
Dx:	RPR → FTA antibodies Lumbar Puncture
Tx:	Penicillin IV Desensitize if penicillin allergic NEVER tetracycline
Baby:	1st Trimester: Fetal Loss 3rd Trimester: Saddle Nose, Saber Shins, Hutchinson's Teeth

HIV	
Path:	Infects baby during birth, not gestation
Pt:	Opportunistic infections Asx Screen
Dx:	ELISA Screen Western Blot Confirm 4th Gen ab-ag tests CD4 + Viral Load
Tx:	Zidovudine-based HAART
PPx:	AZT during birth
F/u:	ELISA not effective for 6 months on baby; mom's antibodies cross placenta, get HIV PCR No breastfeeding

OB

OB Operations

METHOD	INDICATION	MODIFIERS	SIDE EFFECTS
C-Section	Fetal Distress - Nonreassuring CST - Breech Birth - Fetal Bradycardia	Os not @ 10 cm	↑ Risk of rupture with attempted VBAC
	Maternal Distress - PreE, Eclampsia - Hemorrhage	Station ≤ 0	Repeat pregnancy after C-section < 2 C-sections and Low transverse cut - Try Vaginal Deliver - If it works = VBAC = Best outcome - If it doesn't = TOLAC = worst outcome
	Elective - Pfannenstiel = Bikini - Low transverse	Contractions Irrelevant	> 2 C-sections or classical cut - Planned C-section - TOLAC worse, VBAC Better
Forceps	Fetal Distress Prolonged Labor	Os @ 10 cm Station ≥ +1	Facial Palsy Cephalohematoma
Vacuum	Fetal Distress Prolonged Labor	Os @ 10 cm Station ≥ +1	Vaginal Bleeding Denuding of Vagina
Episiotomy	Macrosomic babies in nulliparous moms Prolonged labor Prevent uncontrolled lacerations	Medial Mediolateral	∅ heals, ∅ Hurts, Grade IV Heals, Hurts, no grade IV
Cerclage	Recurrent second trimester losses Incompetent Cervix	Place week 12-14 Remove week 36-38	ppROM (you nick baby 12-16 wks) Cervical Rupture (fail to remove 34-38 wks)
Anesthesia	Narcotics		Naloxone for baby
	Paracervical block	Pain of cervical dilation Local Lidocaine	Fetal bradycardia rarely, NOT an indication for section
	Pudendal Block	Ischial tuberosity Sacrospinous Ligament	You can miss
	Epidural	Preferred method for delivery and C/S	Into CSF = shock

Contraception

EFFECTIVE AND INVASIVE			NONINVASIVE AND EFFECTIVE			NONINVASIVE NOT EFFECTIVE	
Nexplanon	Implantable	3 years	Depo-Provera	IM	3 months	Male Condoms	STD protection
IUD - Mirena - Copper	Implantable	5 years	Orthoevra Nuvaring	Patch	↑↑ DVT/PE	Female Diaphragms	
				Vaginal ring	Falls Out		
Tubal Ligation	Surgical	Irreversible	OCPs	Daily Pill	Daily Compliance	Female Condom	STD Protection
Vasectomy	Surgical	Irreversible	MiniPill (Progestin)	Daily Pill	Strict Compliance		

** LARC (IUDs, especially copper) have been shown to the most effective form of contraception for all age groups and are approved for adolescents, adults, nulliparous, multiparous, etc. They are the best option for long-term contraception (over OCPs AND over tubal ligation).

** Emergency contraception can be either Plan B or an IUD

*** > 35 year old, smoker, and hormones = DVT/PE

**** DO NOT WORK = Family Planning, Withdrawal, Spermicide

Pre-Op Evaluation

CARDIAC	
Pt:	Heart Failure, EF < 35% Myocardial Infarct within 6 months Goldman Index (outdated for pre-op evaluation, but good marker)
Dx:	ECG, Echo, Cath
Tx:	Stenting + Plavix, CABG, Medical Management = BB, ACE-I, ASA, Statin

METABOLIC STATUS	
Path:	DON'T DO SURGERY IF THERE IS DKA
Pt:	Diabetic with elevated blood glucose
Dx:	Check a sugar
Tx:	IVF + Insulin

PULMONARY	
Path:	Ventilation is more an issue than Oxygen
Pt:	Smokers, COPD/Asthma, ILD
Dx:	PFTs for diagnosis ABG showing low O_2 bad, high CO_2 worse
Tx:	Smoking cessation, but only 8 weeks before surgery, quitting closer to surgery makes it worse

LIVER (CHILD-PUGH)	
Path:	Assesses how well the patient can process anesthesia
Pt:	For Child-Pugh (Class A, B, or C) Albumin (low) PT/PTT (elevations) Bilirubin (elevations) Ascites Encephalopathy
Dx:	For MELD score use the equation (do not memorize this equation) Most Surgeries contraindicated in cirrhosis
Tx:	Liver transplant

NUTRITION	
Path:	Need adequate nutrition for healing
Pt:	At risk are people who lost 20% of their body weight in 3 months, albumin < 3, or a failed skin Anergy test
Dx:	CRP, Prealbumin to ensure low albumin is from nutrition Skin Anergy test
Tx:	PO > IV 10 days > 5 days

Post-op Fever

MALIGNANT HYPERTHERMIA (WONDER DRUGS)	
Time:	During Surgery
Tx:	Dantrolene, Cooling, O_2
PPx:	Family History

BACTEREMIA (WOUND)	
Time:	Right After Surgery (post-op day 0)
Tx:	Blood culture, antibiotics
PPx:	Don't poke the bowel

ATELECTASIS (WIND)	
Time:	Day 1
Tx:	CXR, Incentive Spirometer
PPx:	Spirometer

PNEUMONIA (WIND)	
Time:	Day 2
Tx:	Abx → Vanc + Pip/Tazo for HAP
PPx:	Spirometer

UTI (WATER)	
Time:	Day 3
Tx:	Urinalysis (leuk esterase, nitrites, bacteria but no epithelial cells Antibiotics
PPx:	Remove catheter early

DEEP VEIN THROMBOSIS (WALKING)	
Time:	Day 5
Tx:	Ultrasound, Heparin → Warfarin
PPx:	Ambulation, Heparin

WOUND (WOUND)	
Time:	Day 7
Tx:	Cellulitis is visible Ultrasound (r/o abscess), Antibiotics
PPx:	Don't mess up your surgeries

ABSCESS	
Time:	Day 10
Tx:	CT scan, Drain, Antibiotics
PPx:	Don't mess up your surgeries!

Chest Pain

MYOCARDIAL INFARCTION	
Path:	Atherosclerosis
Pt:	Post-op, Silent MI, noticed on ECG
Dx:	ECG, Troponins
Tx:	MONA-BASH, PCI Try ~~tPa~~ (Never tPa post-op!)

DEEP VEIN THROMBOSIS / PULMONARY EMBOLISM	
Path:	Post-op patients are bed-ridden, just had manipulation, highest risk in ortho patients
Pt:	Pleuritic Chest Pain, signs/symptoms of DVT
Dx:	U/S of the legs CT Spiral Chest or V/Q Scan
Tx:	Heparin drip → Warfarin IVC filter only if there is a reason for no anticoagulation

Altered Mental Status

ELECTROLYTES	
Path:	We control feeding, electrolytes, fluid
Pt:	AMS
Dx:	BMP
Tx:	Na, Ca replacement

HYPOXIA	
Path:	Atelectasis, Pain of post-op, underlying dz
Pt:	AMS low sat
Dx:	Pulse Oximetry ABG
Tx:	Oxygen, Incentive Spirometry

ARDS	
Path:	Noncardiogenic pulmonary edema
Pt:	Tumultuous course in the ICU
Dx:	CXR shows white out
Tx:	PEEP (see pulmonology—ARDS)

DELIRIUM TREMENS	
Path:	Alcohol Withdrawal
Pt:	48-72 hrs after admission, hypertension, tachycardia, diaphoretic, hallucinations
Dx:	Clinical
Tx:	Benzodiazepines
PPx:	Long-acting benzos

Abdominal Distention

PARALYTIC ILEUS	
Path:	Metabolic, K
Pt:	Days following surgery, no gas, no stool
Dx:	KUB shows small bowel and large bowel both distended
Tx:	Moving, Eating, Fix potassium

OBSTRUCTION	
Path:	Adhesions (previous surgery) Hernias (no previous surgery)
Pt:	"Ileus" continues to day 5
Dx:	KUB shows dilation / air-fluid levels proximal to the obstruction, collapsed bowel distal to that, Either SBO or LBO, not both
Tx:	NG Tube decompression Surgery

OGILVIE'S (PSEUDO-OBSTRUCTION)	
Path:	Ileus of the elderly
Pt:	Elderly patient, bed bound, nursing home Nontender but very distended
Dx:	KUB shows dilation of the ENTIRE large bowel, but small bowel is normal
Tx:	Rectal Tube Pyridostigmine

Wound

DEHISCENCE	
Path:	Failure of the fascia
Pt:	Hernia, Serosanguinous drainage (salmon colored)
Dx:	Clinical
Tx:	Bind, limit straining Electively to the OR

EVISCERATION	
Path:	Failure of the fascia AND skin, failure of the whole wound
Pt:	Loops of bowel are falling out of the wound
Dx:	Clinical
Tx:	Warm Saline Dressing, Bed Rest EMERGENTLY to the OR

Fistula

FISTULA	
F	Foreign Body
E	Epithelialization
T	Tumor
I	Irradiation / Inflammation / IBD
D	Distal Obstruction
	Remove the Fistula (LIFT procedure)

OR

FISTULA	
F	Foreign Body
R	Radiation
I	Inflammation / Infection
E	Epithelialization
N	Neoplasm
D	Distal Obstruction
	Remove the Fistula (LIFT procedure)

Decreased Urinary Output

URINARY RETENTION	
Path:	Post-op "ileus" of the ureter / urethra vs. BPH
Pt:	Has the urge to void
Dx:	In-and-out cath (post-void residual)
Tx:	Foley cath if unable to void on own

ZERO URINE OUTPUT	
Path:	Kinked Foley
Pt:	Patient has 0 urine output
Dx:	Unkink / flush Foley, watch it dump into bag
Tx:	Unkink / flush Foley, watch it dump into bag

OTHER RENAL FAILURE	
Path:	Prerenal, Postrenal, Intrarenal
Pt:	Post-op patients with normal renal function to start almost always are volume down because of NPO
Dx:	500 cc fluid challenge
Tx:	If improves, continue fluid, if not, check out the renal failure videos in nephrology.

Obstructive Jaundice

TYPES OF JAUNDICE	
Prehepatic	Unconjugated, Hemolysis / Hematoma
Intrahepatic	Mixed, Genetic, Hepatitis
Posthepatic	Conjugated, Obstruction

PAINFUL JAUNDICE	
Path:	Gallstones (choledocolithiasis)
Pt:	Fever, Leukocytosis, Jaundice, Pain,
Dx:	RUQ Ultrasound = biliary duct dilation (choledocolithiasis) MRCP
Tx:	ERCP (also best diagnostic test)

PAINLESS JAUNDICE	
Path:	Cancer, Stricture, PSC
Pt:	Painless jaundice, no fever, no leukocytosis, Courvoisier's sign (distended palpable, painless gallbladder)
Dx:	1st: Ultrasound = thin walled, distended gallbladder Then: ERCP vs. EUS (depending on the cancer)
Tx:	Stage with CT, Resection

PANCREATIC ADENOCARCINOMA	
Path:	Cancer of the head of the pancreas
Pt:	Weight loss, clay colored stools, painless jaundice, migratory thrombophlebitis
Dx:	1st: CT scan Best: EUS with Biopsy
Tx:	Stage with CT Pancreatoduodenectomy (Whipple's)

CHOLANGIOCARCINOMA	
Path:	Cancer of the biliary tree
Pt:	Weight loss, clay stools, painless jaundice
Dx:	ERCP with Biopsy
Tx:	Resection vs. Stenting

CANCER OF AMPULLA OF VATER	
Path:	Cancer that blocks the lumen of the biliary tree that exits into the duodenum
Pt:	Weight loss, clay stools, painless jaundice, fecal occult blood tests
Dx:	ERCP with Biopsy
Tx:	Resection

PRIMARY SCLEROSING CHOLANGITIS	
Path:	Autoimmune disease, men
Pt:	Ulcerative Colitis and painless, obstructive jaundice
Dx:	1st: MRCP (beads on a string) Best: ERCP with biopsy (not needed if MRCP positive)
Tx:	Ursodeoxycholic acid for symptoms ~~STENT~~ (complicates transplant) Transplant
F/u:	See Medicine: GI, Cirrhosis

BILIARY STRICTURES	
Path:	Inflammation or previous endoscopy, stenting
Pt:	Painless jaundice, usually without weight loss
Dx:	MRCP then ERCP
Tx:	Stenting

Esophagus

GERD	
Path:	Lower esophageal sphincter fails, acid reflux
Pt:	Esophageal burning, worse with lying flat and spicy foods, better with sitting upright and with antacids Nocturnal asthma
Dx:	No alarm symptoms: Lifestyle + PPI Alarm symptoms: EGD with Bx
Tx:	GERD: PPIs Metaplasia: ↑ PPI + ↑ Surveillance Dysplasia: Cryoablation Adenocarcinoma: Esophagectomy Nissen Fundoplication

BOERHAAVE'S	
Path:	Transmural tear, Air in the mediastinum
Pt:	Alcoholic, Bulimic Mediastinitis: fever and leukocytosis
Dx:	1st: Gastrografin Then: Barium swallow Best: EGD (only if others are negative)
Tx:	Surgery

ACHALASIA	
Path	LES fails to relax
Pt:	Knot or ball of food gets stuck
Dx:	Barium swallow = bird's beak esophagus Manometry = tight LES
Tx:	Myotomy Dilation, Botox (inferior to Myotomy)
F/u:	GERD if too much

ESOPHAGEAL CANCER	
Path:	↑ 1/3 = SCC 2/2 Hot drinks, smoking ↓ 1/3 = Adeno 2/2 GERD
Pt:	Dysphagia, Odynophagia, Weight Loss
Dx:	Barium Swallow (localizes cancer) EGD with Bx
Tx:	Resection = Esophagectomy

MALLORY-WEISS	
Path:	Superficial tear
Pt:	Self-limiting UGIB Weekend warriors who vomit a lot
Dx:	None needed
Tx:	Self-limiting
F/u:	If continued bleeding, however, treat it like a UGIB . . . NG tube, EGD, 2 large-bore IVs, Type and Cross, transfuse prn

Small Bowel

SMALL BOWEL OBSTRUCTION	
Path:	Adhesions (if previous GI surgery) Hernias (if NO previous GI surgery)
Pt:	Colicky Abdominal Pain Flatus and Bowel Movements → Obstipation Borborygmi → Absent
Dx:	1st: Upright KUB = Air-Fluid Levels Then: CT scan gastrografin po contrast
Tx:	Complete Obstruction: Go to Surgery Incomplete: NG Tube decompression . . . Wait 3 days . . . go to surgery if no change Peritoneal Signs: Straight to surgery

CARCINOID	
Path:	Produces Serotonin, must metastasize to liver to produce symptoms
Pt:	Flushing, wheezing, diarrhea, right sided fibrosis of the tricuspid valve
Dx:	5-HIAA in the urine Octreotide Scan CT scan
Tx:	Resection Octreotide injections

HERNIAS	
Path:	Different hernias have different pathology Direct Hernias: Adults, Transversalis, Inguinal Hernias, Males Indirect: Babies, Patent processus vaginalis, Inguinal Ring, Inguinal Hernia Femoral: Women, under the inguinal ligament Ventral: postoperative, iatrogenic, failure of fascial plane
Pt:	Abdominal Bulge
Dx:	Physical Exam
Tx:	Depends on severity - Reducible: Elective Repair - Incarcerated: Urgent Repair - Strangulated: Emergent Repair

APPENDICITIS	
Path:	Fecalith, Transmural Necrosis, Perforation
Pt:	Umbilical pain that will disappear and then return at McBurney's point, with nausea and anorexia
Dx:	NONE NEEDED CT scan if equivocal
Tx:	Surgery

Pancreas

ACUTE PANCREATITIS	
Path:	Alcohol and Gallstones
Pt:	Epigastric pain that bores to the back Positional Chest pain, nausea, vomiting
Dx:	↑ Amylase, ↑ Lipase You DON'T need a CT scan
Tx:	NPO, IVF, Analgesia
F/u:	CT scan if and only if no improvement

CHRONIC PANCREATITIS	
Path:	Repeated Acute pancreatitis
Pt:	Chronic Pain Similar to Acute Pancreatitis
Dx:	CT scan . . . Lipase can be NORMAL
Tx:	Pain control DO NOT do surgery

NECROTIZING PANCREATITIS	
Path:	Severe Pancreatitis
Pt:	Poor Ranson's Criteria Falling hemoglobin Deteriorating patient DAYS after initial presentation
Dx:	CT scan Biopsy (no abx without proven infxn)
Tx:	Meropenem Serial CTs ICU Surgical Drainage / Debridement

PANCREATIC ABSCESS	
Path:	Infection with the pancreas
Pt:	Fever, leukocytosis that fails to resolve DAYS after pancreatitis
Dx:	CT scan
Tx:	Antibiotics, IR Drainage vs. Surgery vs. Endoscopic

PSEUDOCYSTS	
Path:	Fluid filled vesicle that is NOT lined by endothelium
Pt:	Early satiety, ascites, dyspnea WEEKS after pancreatitis
Dx:	CT scan
Tx:	< 6 cm and < 6 weeks = watch and wait ≥ 6 cm or > 6 weeks = Drain either Surgery (percutaneous) or Endoscopic (gastric, duodenum)

Leg Ulcers

COMPRESSION ULCERS	
Path:	Pressure points
Pt:	Bed-ridden patients who don't move. Ulcers occur on shoulders, elbows, sacrum, ankles, knees . . . constitutes abuse
Dx:	Clinical
Tx:	Rolling Getting out of bed Air mattress

DIABETIC ULCERS	
Path:	Neuropathy, microvascular
Pt:	Diabetic Ulcers occur on Heels and toes
Dx:	Clinical
Tx:	Control blood glucose Wound clean Amputation

ARTERIAL INSUFFICIENCY	
Path:	No blood going in

Pt:	Peripheral Vascular Disease
	   - Hairless leg
	   - Decreased pulses
	   - Scaly legs
	Ulcers at tips of toes . . . dry gangrene

Dx:	Ankle Brachial Index Ultrasound with Doppler Arteriogram
Tx:	Stent vs. Bypass Amputation Smoking cessation

VENOUS STASIS ULCER	
Path:	No blood going out
Pt:	Edema, hyperpigmentation, Indurated Medial Malleolus
Dx:	Clinical
Tx:	Control → CHF / Nephrotic / Cirrhosis Compression Stockings, Unna Boots

MARJOLIN'S ULCER	
Path:	SCC
Pt:	Wound repeatedly healing and breaking down with a continuous draining tract Ulcer = Ugly, Deep, Heaped margins
Dx:	Punch biopsy
Tx:	Wide resection

Colorectal

COLON CANCER	
Path:	Right sided bleed, but do not obstruct Left sided do not bleed, but do obstruct
Pt:	Post-Menopausal Female or any Male with iron deficiency anemia Alternating bowel habits with change in the caliber of the stool
Dx:	Colonoscopy
Tx:	CT scan to stage Resection Chemo (FOLFOX, FOLFIRI)
PPx:	Screening Colonoscopy

FAMILIAL ADENOMATOUS POLYPOSIS	
Path:	Genetic
Pt:	1000s of polyps by 20 Cancer by 30 Death by 40
Dx:	Colonoscopy
Tx:	Prophylactic Colectomy

POLYP	
Path:	Pedunculated, Small, Tubular = Benign Sessile, Large, Villous = Worrisome
Pt:	Asymptomatic = screening colonoscopy
Dx:	Colonoscopy with biopsy
Tx:	No polyp = 10 years Benign Polyp = 5-7 years Premalignant = 3-5 years Carcinoma in Situ = 1-3 years

ULCERATIVE COLITIS	
Path:	Autoimmune—Ashkenazi Jews Superficial Colitis
Pt:	Bloody bowel movement + weight loss Associated with PSC Associated with Seronegative Arthritis
Dx:	Colonoscopy = continuous lesions Biopsy = superficial inflammation
Tx:	Resection (before cancer) Can try monoclonal antibody anti-TNF
F/u:	> 8 years from diagnosis, MANDATORY annual colonoscopies, RECOMMENDED prophylactic colectomy

FISTULA	
Path:	Crohn's Disease, Transmural inflammation, Local Radiation Endothelial-lined connection from any two organs GI tract to anything (vagina, skin, bladder)
Pt:	Fecal Soiling
Dx:	Probing
Tx:	LIFT = Fistulotomy

HEMORRHOIDS	
Path:	Internal—bleed, but do not hurt External—hurt, but do not bleed
Pt:	Dark blood on the toilet paper after BM, rectal pain, tenesmus
Dx:	Visual Inspection
Tx:	High-fiber diet Internal—Banded External—Removed (resection) Sitz baths, Preparation H (usually fails)

ANAL FISSURES	
Path:	Tight sphincter
Pt:	Pain on defecation that lasts for hours, fear of defecation
Dx:	Visual inspection
Tx:	Sitz baths, nitroglycerin paste, calcium channel blocker paste, Botox injection Lateral Internal Sphincterotomy

ANAL CANCER	
Path:	Squamous Cell Carcinoma secondary to HPV
Pt:	Anoreceptive Sex, men with men HIV positive Anal Pap
Dx:	Biopsy
Tx:	Chemo and Radiation (Nigro Protocol) Usually resection is NOT needed
F/u:	Assess for HIV if status not known

Colorectal

PILONIDAL CYST	
Path:	Abscessed Hair Follicle
Pt:	Congenital Defect Hairy Butt
Dx:	Clinical (tract with hair upon incision and drainage)
Tx:	Incision and Drainage Resection of the Cyst

Breast Cancer

BREAST CANCER	
Path:	Estrogen—Obesity, Nulliparity, Early Menarche, Late Menopause, HRT Genes—BRCA1/2, Radiation
Pt:	Asymptomatic Screen Breast Lump, Breast Mass
Dx:	Mammogram Core Needle Biopsy

Tx:	Lumpectomy + radiation = Mastectomy Sentinel Lymph Node Biopsy Axillary Lymph Node Dissection if positive Chemo
	  - HER2/neu +
	    - Trastuzumab
	  - ER/PR +
	    - Tamoxifen (pre-meno-pausal)
	    - Anastrozole (post-meno-pausal)
	  - All
	    - Doxorubicin or Daunoru-bicin (anthracycline) based regimen

BREAST CANCER SCREEN	
USPTF:	50q2, start at 50, every 2 years
ACS:	40q1, start at 40, every 1 year
All:	Mammogram → Core Needle Biopsy
BRCA:	MRI

DIAGNOSTIC DILEMMA: THE YOUNG WOMAN	
	< 30 gets a different set of rules
Then Then Then	< 30 = Reassurance x 2-3 cycles < 30 + persists = Ultrasound < 30 + cyst on ultrasound = FNA < 30 + cyst resolves = reassurance
OR OR OR	Mammogram and Core Needle Biopsy if . . . > 30 Ultrasound shows mass Aspirate is bloody Cyst recurs after aspiration

PICK THE TREATMENT	
Local Disease:	Surgical Therapy Lumpectomy + Radiation <u>OR</u> Mastectomy Sentinel Lymph Node Biopsy and then Axillary Lymph Node Dissection if +
Spread Disease:	Systemic Therapy Chemo: Doxorubicin, Paclitaxel HER2/neu: Trastuzumab ER/PR: SERMS (premenopausal) ER/PR: Aromatase-I (postmenopausal)

KNOW YOUR TREATMENTS	
Tamoxifen:	Better, ↑ DVT, ↑ Endo Ca
Raloxifene:	Worse, ↓ DVT, ↓ Endo Ca
Trastuzumab:	Heart Failure, Reversible, EARLY
Doxorubicin:	Heart Failure, Irreversible, LATE
Daunorubicin:	The other Doxorubicin
ALND:	Sentinel Lymph Node First

Pediatrics First Day

ESOPHAGEAL ATRESIA	
Path:	Atresia of the esophagus May or may not be fistula to trachea
Pt:	Coughing and choking with feeds Gurgling or Bubbling
Dx:	NG Tube placed = coiled in esophagus
Tx:	Surgery . . .BUT . . .
F/u:	**VACTERL** = Vertebral, Anus, Cardiac, Trachea, Esophagus, Renal, Limb

IMPERFORATE ANUS	
Path:	Atretic Colon
Pt:	No hole at anus NEVER take first temp rectally!
Dx:	Up-side-down babygram (X-ray)
Tx:	Small distance = fix now Large Distance = Colostomy and fix before toilet training begins

CONGENITAL DIAPHRAGMATIC HERNIA	
Path:	Failure of fusion of diaphragm Posterior (Bochdalek) > Lateral (Morgagni) Crushed developing lung = hypoplastic lung
Pt:	Bowel sounds in the chest Scaphoid abdomen
Dx:	X-ray (babygram) = Bowel in the chest
Tx:	Surgery for the hernia Intubation and surfactant for the hypoplastic lung . . . high ventilatory rate

GASTROSCHISIS	
Path:	Failure of bowel development Inability to reenter abdomen
Pt:	Lesion to the right of midline WITHOUT a membrane
Dx:	Clinical (bowel is hanging out of baby)
Tx:	Silo

OMPHALOCELE	
Path	Failure of bowel development Inability to reenter the abdomen
Pt:	Midline lesion contained by a membrane
Dx:	Clinical (bowel is hanging out)
Tx:	Silo

ANNULAR PANCREAS	
Path:	Migrating branch of pancreas fails to undergo apoptosis
Pt:	Bilious vomiting with double bubble
Dx:	Babygram shows double bubble ONLY
Tx:	Resection of extra pancreas segment

INTESTINAL ATRESIA	
Path:	Intrauterine vascular accident Mom did cocaine
Pt:	Bilious vomiting with double bubble
Dx:	Babygram—multiple air fluid levels
Tx:	Resection of atretic segments

MALROTATION	
Path:	Bowel twisting on its own vascular supply
Pt:	Bilious vomiting with double bubble
Dx:	X-ray (babygram) = normal gas pattern beyond Air or Contrast Enema Upper GI series if enema negative
Tx:	Emergent Surgical Intervention

NECROTIZING ENTEROCOLITIS	
Path:	Premature Neonate disease
Pt:	Preemie with bloody bowel movement after first feed Abdominal distention and ↓ platelets
Dx:	Babygram shows pneumatosis intestinalis
Tx:	NPO, TPN
F/u:	Watch out for other premature diseases: - Intraventricular Hemorrhage - Retinopathy of prematurity - Bronchopulmonary Dysplasia

Pediatrics Weeks to Months

MECONIUM ILEUS	
Path:	Cystic fibrosis
Pt:	Failure to pass meconium Bilious emesis
Dx:	1st: Babygram = ground-glass loops of bowel Best: Barium-Enema
Tx:	Barium-Enema (also treatment)

PYLORIC STENOSIS	
Path:	Hypertrophied pylorus creates an effective gastric outlet obstruction
Pt:	Male baby, projectile vomiting after eating Visible Peristalsis, 4-8 weeks old Olive-shaped mass in abdomen
Dx:	Ultrasound shows the donut sign
Tx:	Myotomy
F/u:	Fix electrolytes before surgery, that is usually the "next step" Hypochloremic Hypokalemic Metabolic Alkalosis

BILIARY ATRESIA	
Path:	Biliary tree is atretic
Pt:	Persistent jaundice (conjugated)
Dx:	HIDA scan 1 week after phenobarbital
Tx:	Resection of atretic segments

HIRSCHSPRUNG'S	
Path:	Failure of neurons to migrate into the colon Absence of Auerbach plexus
Pt:	Failure to pass meconium at day #1 Chronic diarrhea at any age
Dx:	KUB /Babygram = distended good bowel, normal looking bad bowel
Tx:	Remove bad segment

INTUSSUSCEPTION	
Path:	Telescoping of bowel into itself leading to vascular compromise May be caused by Meckel's diverticulum
Pt:	Abdominal pain Fetal position Currant-Jelly Diarrhea
Dx:	1st: KUB = sausage-shaped mass Best: Air enema
Tx:	Air enema Resection of dead bowel

Surgical Hypertension

PRIMARY HYPERALDOSTERONISM (CONN'S)	
Path:	Tumor of adrenal gland = aldosterone
Pt:	Hypertension and Hypokalemia
Dx:	1st: Aldosterone: Renin ratio > 20 CT scan If not sure . . . adrenal vein sampling
Tx:	Resection

RENAL ARTERY STENOSIS	
Pt:	Old Man: Atherosclerosis of renal artery Young Female: Fibromuscular Dysplasia
Dx:	1st: Aldosterone: Renin ratio < 10 Then: U/S Doppler shows gradient drop Best: Arteriogram
Tx:	Fibromuscular Dysplasia = Stenting Old man with RAS = medical management means high dose ACE-I / ARBS or Aldosterone Antagonists

PHEOCHROMOCYTOMA	
Path:	Catecholamine excess May be part of the MEN syndromes
Pt:	Paroxysms Pressure Pain Palpitations Perspirations
Dx:	24-hour urinary VMA and metanephrines MIBG scan
Tx:	α-blockade then β-blockade, then resection

COARCTATION OF AORTA	
Path:	Congenital Disease
Pt:	Torso high blood pressure, legs have low blood pressure Child: pain on walking, refuses to walk Adult: rib notching, HTN, cold legs
Dx:	1st: X-ray = notching CT or MR angiogram Arteriogram (not needed)
Tx:	Resection of coarctation with reanastomosis

Endocrine see medicine for more details

THYROID NODULE	
Pt:	Nodule in the neck
Dx:	1st: TSH/FT4 Then: RAIU Best: Biopsy = FNA
Tx:	If hyperthyroid, RAIU hot, noncancerous, go to iodine ablation, surgical resection If euthyroid, RAIU cold, biopsy, cancerous go to surgical resection with staging or iodine ablation if follicular carcinoma

GLUCAGONOMA	
Path:	Glucagon secreted from pancreas
Pt:	Necrolytic Migratory Erythema Diabetes
Dx:	↑ Glucagon ~~Glucose fails to suppress glucagon~~ CT scan
Tx:	Resection

1° HYPERPARATHYROIDISM	
Path:	Too much parathyroid hormone
Pt:	Hyper Ca, Hypo Phos, Hyper PTH Hyper Ca = Bones, Stones, groans
Dx:	Sestamibi scan
Tx:	Resection of parathyroid glands
F/u:	Hypocalcemia following surgery

ZOLLINGER-ELLISON	
Path:	Gastrin secreting tumor
Pt:	Multiple, severe ulcers refractory to treatment with diarrhea
Dx:	Gastrin in the 1000s Somatostatin Suppression test shows a paradoxical ↑ Gastrin Somatostatin Receptor Scintigraphy (localization)
Tx:	Resection

INSULINOMA	
Path:	Extra insulin is secreted from the pancreas
Pt:	Repeated hypoglycemia especially when fasting, may present as syncope
Dx:	72 hour fast and then, with symptoms, check: - Blood Glucose (confirm low bG) - C-Peptide (r/o malingering) - Sulfonylurea Screen (r/o malingering)
Tx:	CT scan to see the tumor Resection

Endocrine

Cushing's in General	
Path:	Excess Cortisol Pills, Pituitary, Adrenal, Ectopic Tumor
Pt:	Women with HTN and DM . . . AND . . . Central Obesity, Buffalo Hump, Moon Facies

Dx:	"LOW THEN HIGH"
	- **Low** Dose Dexa Suppression test
	(confirm 24-hour urine cortisol)
	   - AC**THen**
	   - **High**-Dose Dexa Suppression
	     Test
	MRI if in the brain
	CT scan of the abdomen

Tx:	Resection of lesion Taper Steroids if that's the cause

Cushing's—Cushing's DISEASE	
Path:	Pituitary tumor, ACTH-dependent
Pt:	Cushing's
Dx:	1st: Low-Dose Dexa = Fails to Suppress Then: ACTH = High Then: High-dose Dexa Suppresses Then: MRI Then: Inferior Petrosal Sinus Sampling
Tx:	Pituitary resection vs. radiation

Cushing's—Ectopic Tumor	
Path:	Lung Tumor (small cell), ACTH- dependent
Pt:	Cushing's
Dx:	1st: Low-Dose Dexa = Fails to Suppress Then: ACTH = High Then: High-dose Dexa: Fails to Suppress Then: CT scan of Chest/Abd/Pelvis = Tumor
Tx:	Tumor resection

Cushing's—Primary Hypercortisolism	
Path:	Pituitary Tumor, ACTH-Independent
Pt:	Cushing's
Dx:	1st: Low-Dose Dexa = Fails to Suppress Then: ACTH = Low CT scan abd = tumor
Tx:	Resection

CT Surgery

AORTIC STENOSIS	
Path:	Calcification, Atherosclerosis, Bicuspid valve
Pt:	Old man with chest pain (most common) Syncope, CHF (worse) 2nd intercostal space, right sternal border with systolic crescendo-decrescendo murmur Radiates to clavicle / carotid
Dx:	Echocardiogram
Tx:	Replacement ~~Valvotomy~~ (never the right answer) TAVR or TAVI if not good surgical candidate
F/u:	LHC first, may need CABG in addition to valve replacement INR 2.5-3.5 post replacement

AORTIC REGURGITATION	
Path:	Infection, Infarction, Dissection
Pt:	Acute (devastating, shock, very fast) Chronic (insidious, murmur only) 2nd intercostal space right sternal border diastolic decrescendo murmur Widened Pulse Pressure Water Hammer Pulses Pistol Shot Pulses Head-bobbing
Dx:	Echocardiogram
Tx:	~~Intra-aortic balloon pump~~ (contraindicated) Replacement
F/u:	LHC first, may need CABG

MITRAL STENOSIS	
Path:	Rheumatic Heart Disease
Pt:	Apex of the heart (5th intercostal space) Diastolic rumbling with opening snap AFib, CHF
Dx:	Echocardiogram
Tx:	Medically Manage until patient ready Balloon Valvotomy ~~Commissurotomy~~ (not done anymore) Eventual replacement

MITRAL REGURGITATION	
Path:	Infection, Infarction
Pt:	Papillary rupture > Chordae Tendinae Holosystolic murmur that radiates to the axilla, obscures underlying heart sounds
Dx:	Echocardiogram
Tx:	Replacement

CORONARY ARTERY DISEASE = CABG	
Path:	Obese, HTN, Diabetic, Smoker, Dyslipidemia
Pt:	Left Sided, substernal chest pain Worse with exertion, better with rest Relieved with Nitro
Dx:	ECG → STEMI Troponins → NSTEMI Stress Test → Coronary Artery Disease Angiogram → # of vessels and distribution
Tx:	1 Vessel disease = Stent + Clopidogrel 3+ Vessels = CABG Left Mainstem = CABG Internal Mammary to the most important vessel (often the largest) Saphenous Vein grafting to other vessels
F/u:	Reinfarction in hospital use CKMB, NOT troponin—troponin will be elevated post-surgery Reinfarction caught by ECG . . . NOT chest pain—all post-op hearts have chest pain, their chest was cracked open Medical management = aspirin, statin, β-blocker, ACE-inhibitor, clopidogrel, and risk factor management

Pediatrics CT

LEFT TO RIGHT SHUNTS
↑ Pulmonary Flow
↑ Pulmonary Vasculature on X-ray
↑ Pulmonary Pressures
Right Ventricular Hypertrophy
Eisenmenger's (reversal to Right to Left)
"D" Diseases: ASD, VSD, PDA

ATRIAL SEPTAL DEFECT	
Path:	Ostium Primum (rare) Ostium Secundum (more common)
Pt:	Fixed Split S2 Most Common Murmur > 1 year old
Dx:	Echo
Tx:	Surgical closure

VENTRICULAR SEPTAL DEFECT	
Path:	Hole between the two ventricles
Pt:	Harsh Holosystolic Murmur in a neonate . . . but the worst defects have no murmur Most common congenital heart disease . . . but they get fixed or die before 1 year Failure to thrive, Down's Syndrome
Dx:	Echo
Tx:	If CHF, Failure to thrive, dyspnea = fix now If none of those things = fix before year 1, may resolved spontaneously
F/u:	Surgical closure required before the end of year 1 in all cases

PATENT DUCTUS ARTERIOSUS	
Path:	Ductus arteriosus remains open, a connection between aorta and pulmonary artery
Pt:	Continuous Machinery-Like Murmur
Dx:	Echo
Tx:	If no CHF → Indomethacin = Ends the PDA If yes CHF → Surgical Closure If Tetralogy → prostaglandins to sustain PDA
F/u:	All PDAs must be closed before 8 mo.

Truncus Arteriosus, Tricuspid Atresia, and Total Anomalous Pulmonary Venous Return are intentionally NOT included in this section because they are too low yield for Step 2.

RIGHT TO LEFT SHUNTS
↓ Pulmonary Flow
↓ Pulmonary Vasculature on X-ray
Deoxygenated Blood in periphery
Blue Baby Syndrome
Fatal if not corrected
The "T" Diseases: Tetralogy, TGA, TA, TAPVR

TETRALOGY OF FALLOT	
Path:	1: Overriding Aorta 2: Pulmonary Stenosis 3: Right ventricular Hypertrophy 4: Ventricular Septal Defect "Endocardial Cushion defect"
Pt:	Most common cyanotic disease of children because TGA babies die or get fixed "Tet Spells" cyanosis relieved by squatting
Dx:	1st: Boot Shaped heart on X-ray Best: Echocardiogram
Tx:	Surgical Correction
F/u:	Associated with Down's Syndrome

Pediatrics CT

TRANSPOSITION OF THE GREAT ARTERIES	
Path:	Heart fails to twist Pulmonary Artery and Vein both connected to the left heart and lungs Aorta and Vena Cava both connected to the right heart and periphery TWO separate circulatory systems connected only by ductus arteriosus
Pt:	Blue baby day 1—you will not miss this Mom is a diabetic at the start of pregnancy ~~Gestational Diabetes~~ (not a risk factor)
Dx:	Echo
Tx:	Prostaglandins to support PDA Surgical Correction

COARCTATION OF AORTA	
Path:	Narrowing of aorta, collaterals through rib arteries
Pt:	Hypertension in upper extremities, hypotension in lower extremities in a child Claudication (crying with crawling or walking)
Dx:	Clinical: Blood Pressures in all extremities X-ray shows rib notching (not diagnostic) Aortogram
Tx:	Surgical Correction

Vascular

ABDOMINAL AORTIC ANEURYSM	
Path:	Atherosclerosis Asymptomatic Pulsatile Mass
Pt:	Old Man > 65 who at least ever smoked
Dx:	Screen old men who smoke U/S (preferred) CT scan (allowed) ~~Arteriogram~~ (may look normal)

Tx:	> 5.5 cm or growing > 0.5 cm/year
	   = operate
	< 5.5 cm and growing < 0.5 cm/year
	   = U/S q6

F/u:	Pt with tender pulsatile mass with
	   back pain goes to EMERGENT
	   surgery, the AAA is about to pop

AORTIC DISSECTION	
Path:	Hypertension leads to a . . . Formation of a false lumen Ascending = Great vessels and aortic valve Descending = beyond great vessels
Pt:	Tearing Chest Pain radiating to the back Asymmetric blood pressures left to right arm CXR with a widened mediastinum BONUS: Marfan, Syphilis
Dx:	1st: CXR Best: CT Angiogram ~~Arteriogram~~ (never pick this) . . .If CT not available . . . TEE > MRI

Tx:	Ascending = Type A = Emergent
	   Surgery ± Aortic Valve
	Descending = Type B = Medical
	   Management

ACUTE LIMB ISCHEMIA	
Path:	Cholesterol Emboli—Cath Clot Embolism—AFib Air—Central line
Pt:	**P**ain **P**ulselessness **P**oikilothermic **P**aresthesias **P**ale **P**aralysis
Dx:	1st = Ultrasound with Doppler Best = Arteriogram
Tx:	Intra-arterial tPA Embolectomy Heparin
F/u:	Compartment Syndrome requiring fasciotomy

CHRONIC LIMB ISCHEMIA (PERIPHERAL VASCULAR DZ)	
Path:	Atherosclerosis, Smoking, HTN, DM

Pt:	Claudication (pain in legs on walking)
	   that
	   - Affects lifestyle = investigate
	   - Does not affect lifestyle = no
	      investigation
	Rest Pain (Critical Limb Ischemia)
	   - Scaly Shiny Skin
	   - Hair loss in that extremity
	   - Pain at rest that gets purple and
	      relieved with dependence

Dx:	Ankle-Brachial Index
	   - ≥ 1.2 cm Unable to assess
	   - 0.9 – 1.2 cm Normal
	   - 0.8 – 0.9 cm Mild
	   - 0.5 – 0.8 cm Moderate
	   - < 0.5 cm Severe
	Ultrasound with Doppler
	Arteriogram

Tx:	Treat smoking cessation & exercise to
	   improve collaterals
	Single Lesion
	   - Endovascular Stenting
	      - Femoral
	      - Short Lesions
	   - Bypass Surgery (fem-fem,
	      fem-pop)
	      - Popliteal
	      - ANY long lesion
	Diffuse Disease
	   - Medical management with
	   - Clopidogrel (antiplatelet
	      therapy)
	   - Cilostazol (improves pain)
	Amputation

Adult Ophtho

GLAUCOMA

Path:	Most common cause of blindness Wide Angle: Asymptomatic Narrow Angle: Pain Crisis
Pt:	Patient comes out of low-light situation Pain in the eye, headache, blurry vision Rigid Eyeball, Red, Inflamed Eye
Dx:	Ocular Pressure ↑↑↑
Tx:	Constrict Pupil with α-agonists and β-antagonists Laser to drill a hole NEVER give atropine

PERIORBITAL CELLULITIS

Path:	Inflammation or infection within the orbit No compromise to extraocular muscles No risk to eye loss
Pt:	Fever, Leukocytosis, Inflammation NO extraocular muscle paralysis
Dx:	Clinical diagnosis
Tx:	Antibiotics—strep and staph coverage

ORBITAL CELLULITIS

Path:	Inflammation or infection within the orbit Yes compromise to extraocular muscles Yes risk to eye loss
Pt:	Fever, leukocytosis, inflammation Extraocular muscle paralysis
Dx:	CT scan of max-face
Tx:	Incision and drainage with antibiotics

RETINAL DETACHMENT

Path:	Two ways it can happen: 1. Trauma = MVA 2. Hypertensive emergency
Pt:	"Floaters" = mild disease "Veil or Curtain" = severe disease
Dx:	Ophthalmoscope = Clinical
Tx:	Laser to "spot-weld" the retina back on
F/u:	Spontaneous resolution NOT detachment . . . see Amaurosis Fugax

AMAUROSIS FUGAX

Path:	Impending retinal artery occlusion
Pt:	"Curtain or veil" that comes and goes on its own (retinal detachment doesn't resolve spontaneously like Amaurosis)
Dx:	Otoscope = Clinical
Tx:	HLD, DM, CVA, HTN

RETINAL ARTERY OCCLUSION

Path:	Thrombus or embolism in the retinal artery
Pt:	Painless unilateral loss of vision Without other focal neurologic deficits Previous Amaurosis Fugax
Dx:	Clinical
Tx:	Hyperventilate CO_2 (brown bag) Pressure on globe Intra-arterial tPA if caught early (it is a stroke of the retina)

CORNEAL ABRASION

Path:	Foreign body gets into eye, lacerates the cornea
Pt:	Shop, carpentry, firearms being performed without eye protection Burning eye pain
Dx:	Fluorescein dye
Tx:	Irrigate it a lot Surgery or medical management

Skin Cancer

DISEASE	PHYSICAL	METS	PARANEOPLASTIC	INVASION	DIAGNOSIS	TREATMENT
Basal Cell Carcinoma	Waxy or Pearly	∅ Mets	∅ Paraneoplastic	+ Local Invasion	Incisional Excisional	Resect, Amputate
Squamous Cell Carcinoma	Pigmented or Ulcer	+ Mets	∅ Paraneoplastic	∅ Local Invasion	Incisional Excisional	Resect, Radiation
Melanoma	ABCDE	+ Mets	∅ Paraneoplastic	∅ Local Invasion	Punch Bx Excisional	< 0.5 mm = Local Resect > 1 mm = wide, SNLD > 4 mm = mets, ∅ chemo

BASAL CELL CARCINOMA	
Path:	Basal cells ∅ Metastasize
Pt:	Pearly Lesion Non-healing, bleeds easily Sun-Occupation Sun-Location Sun-People
Dx:	Wide Excisional Biopsy
Tx:	> 1 mm margins on excisions = treated Mohs surgery Amputation of extremity
F/u:	Will locally invade but never metastasizes

SQAUMOUS CELL CARCINOMA	
Path:	Keratinocytes Can, but usually . . . ∅ metastasize
Pt:	Well-demarcated red papules Pigmented lower lip lesion Marjolin ulcer = nonhealing necrotic ulcer that breaks down and flares up again Sun-Occupation Sun-Location Sun-People
Dx:	Wide Excisional Biopsy
Tx:	Same as BCC + Radiation for high risk tumors
F/u:	Skin cancers DO NOT cause paraneoplastic syndromes as other SCC do

DETAILS ABOUT BASAL AND SQUAMOUS CELL DIAGNOSIS	
Dx:	Excisional Biopsy if small and not on face Incisional Biopsy if large OR on face
Tx:	Excisional Biopsy = Small lesion not on face Wide resection = Large lesion not on the face Amputation = Large lesion on extremity Mohs = Any lesion on the face

MELANOMA	
Path:	Melanocytes
Pt:	Jet Black, Smooth lesion Any lesion that is ABCDE (any 1 counts) **A** Asymmetric **B** Border Irregularity **C** Color Mixing **D** Diameter > 5mm **E** Evolving / Changing Sun-Occupation Sun-Location Sun-People
Dx:	~~Shave~~ Punch Biopsy if the lesion is large, on the face, or there is low risk of melanoma Wide Excisional Biopsy is preferred
Tx:	Breslow's depth (in mm) < 0.5: Local resection 1-2: Wide resection, SLND, 1 cm marg 2-4: Wide resection, SLND, 2 cm marg > 4 : Debulking of tumor, palliation
F/u:	Waxes and Wanes naturally Chemo has no benefit Immunotherapy may be a coming therapy

Skin Cancer

RISK OF SKIN CANCER	
Sun-Occupations	Sailor, Farmer, Construction, people who frequent tanning
Sun-Locations	Hands, Face, Back, Shoulders
Sun-People	Fair-skinned, Fair-Haired, and any bad sunburn in their life

Pediatric Ophtho

TYPE	TIME	PURULENT	PROBLEMS	TX
Chemical	24 hrs	Non-purulent	Bilateral	Observation (caused by silver nitrate PPx)
Gonorrhea	Day 2-5	Purulent	Bilateral, Check for systemic illness!	Ceftriaxone IM
Chlamydia	Day 5-14	Muco-purulent	Unilateral then Bilateral Associated with pneumonia	Erythromycin PO No topical antibiotics

RETINOBLASTOMA	
Path:	Rb gene mutation
Pt:	Newborn screen in the neonatal unit with an abnormal light reflex
Dx:	Red reflex (normal) = Pure White Retina "white thing in the BACK of the eye"
Tx:	Surgery Radiation Therapy (NEVER)
F/u:	Osteosarcoma

AMBLYOPIA	
Path:	Cortical Blindness
Pt:	Strabismus, Cataracts, another cause, leads to cortical blindness
Dx:	None
Tx:	None Fix the problem that could lead to cortical blindness

STRABISMUS	
Path:	"Lazy eye"
Pt:	Baby with one eye that focuses while the other does not Almost ALWAYS a photograph question
Dx:	Light reflects at different points on both eyes
Tx:	If present at birth - Patch the good eye - Surgery if all else fails Glasses if developed after birth

CONGENITAL CATARACTS	
Path:	Present at birth → TORCH infections Not present at birth → Galactosemia
Pt:	White cloudy lesions in front of their eye "white thing in FRONT of the eye"
Dx:	Clinical
Tx:	Surgical Removal

RETINOPATHY OF PREMATURITY	
Path:	Premature baby, oxygen toxicity
Pt:	Suspect in any premature neonate especially if any of the "other 3" are present
Dx:	Ophtho Exam = growths on retina
Tx:	Laser Ablation
F/u:	The "other three" Necrotizing Enterocolitis Bronchopulmonary Dysplasia Intraventricular Hemorrhage

This is a duplicate from pediatrics.

Neurosurgery Bleeds

INTRACEREBRAL HEMORRHAGE	
Path:	Hypertension Caudate and putamen most common
Pt:	Focal Neurologic Deficit Headache Coma → death
Dx:	CT scan = Bleed IN the parenchyma
Tx:	SYS BP < 150 ↓ Intracranial Pressure = Hyperventilation Craniotomy VP Shunt

EPIDURAL (SEE TRAUMA)	
Path:	Tearing of middle meningeal artery
Pt:	Walk, talk, and die syndrome following blunt trauma to the head
Dx:	CT scan = Lens-Shaped Hematoma
Tx:	Craniotomy
F/u:	Herniation if not relieved (may require burr hole emergently)

SUBARACHNOID HEMORRHAGE	

Path:	Ruptured aneurysm (anterior
	    communicating artery most
	    common)

Pt:	Thunderclap headache Worst headache of their life Sudden onset headache, maximum intensity Preceded by sentinel bleed

Dx:	CT scan = Blood
	    - Under the arachnoid, outside
	        parenchyma
	    - Fills the cisterns
	LP = Blood / Xanthochromia

Tx:	Coil or Clip within 48 hours or after
	    6 weeks
	Calcium Channel Blocker
	    (vasospasm PPx)
	SYS BP < 150, ↓ ICP

SUBDURAL (SEE TRAUMA)	
Path:	Tearing of bridging veins

Pt:	Acute: young, severe trauma (child
	    abuse) coma to death, "goes out . .
	    . stays out"
	Chronic: old, EtOH, atrophy, fall,
	    with persistent headache and
	    worsening dementia

Dx:	CT scan = crescent shaped hematoma
Tx:	Craniotomy, evacuation

Neurosurgery Tumors

MENINGIOMAS	
Path:	Psammoma Bodies Growth of Dura, not parenchyma
Pt:	Seizures Headache
Dx:	CT Scan shows mass attached to dura
Tx:	Resection
F/u:	No metastasis, does not invade parenchyma, only pushes on

EPENDYMOMA	
Path:	4th Ventricle, Children Ependymal Cells
Pt:	Obstructive Hydrocephalus but there are NO distal cord lesions Curls into fetal position to relieve obstruction symptoms: headache, nausea vomiting
Dx:	MRI
Tx:	Resection

GLIOBLASTOMA MULTIFORME "GBM"	
Path:	Invasive, necrotic, rapidly fatal tumor
Pt:	Focal Neurologic Deficits, Seizure, headache
Dx:	CT Scan shows butterfly lesion Can cross midline
F/u:	Eats brain; permanent deficit, limited prognosis

METASTASIS	
Path:	Primary brain tumors kill before they spread Brain mets from elsewhere usually occur as multiple lesions at grey- white junction
Pt:	Seizures Headache
Dx:	CT Scan shows multiple lesions Look for another cancer
Tx:	Whole brain radiation / Gamma knife to target specific lesions
F/u:	Lung > Prostate/Breast > Colon

MEDULLOBLASTOMA	
Path:	4th Ventricle, Children Highly Malignant
Pt:	Obstructive Hydrocephalus AND distal cord lesions
Dx:	MRI
Tx:	Resection, Chemo, Radiation

Urologic Cancer

RENAL CELL CARCINOMA	
Path:	????
Pt:	Classic Triad: Hematuria, Flank Pain, Palpable Mass Anemia (cancer) OR Polycythemia (EPO)
Dx:	Ultrasound CT scan Nephrectomy (Needle Biopsy)
Tx:	Nephrectomy Chemo . . .

TESTICULAR CANCER	
Path:	Germ cell tumor
Pt:	Painless mass in the scrotum Teenage (15-25)
Dx:	Transillumination (fails to illuminate) Biopsy-FNA (NEVER) Orchiectomy
Tx:	Resection Seminoma—LDH, Chemo + Radiation Endodermal Sinus—AFP Choriocarcinoma—β-hCG Teratoma—Malignant

BLADDER CANCER	
Path:	Smoking, β-alanine dyes
Pt:	Asymptomatic Hematuria Hydronephrosis Hydroureter
Dx:	Ultrasound = Hydro 1st: Cystoscopy Best: Biopsy IVP, VCU
Tx:	Resection Intravesical chemo

PROSTATE CANCER	
Path:	5-DHT (Testosterone)
Pt:	Asymptomatic screen (don't screen PSA) Obstructive Sxs = BPH DRE = Firm + Nodular ↑ PSA
Dx:	1st:PSA (Diagnostic) Best: Biopsy = Transrectal or Transurethral Gleason Score (out of 10, 10 is worst)
Tx:	Surgical resection, Radiation Anti-Androgens (Flutamide) GnRH Analogs (Leuprolide) Orchiectomy (physical androgen deprivation)

Urology Peds

POSTERIOR URETHRAL VALVES	
Path:	Difficulty getting urine out
Pt:	No urine output day 1 of life, elevated creatinine, +/- oligohydramnios
Dx:	Catheter = Residuals Voiding Cystourethrogram
Tx:	Catheter Resection and Reimplant Transplant

EPI/HYPOSPADIAS	
Path:	Ventral—Hypo Dorsal—Epi
Pt:	Has a urethral opening either on the ventral or dorsal surface
Dx:	Clinical
Tx:	NEVER circumcise Rebuild using foreskin

URETEROPELVIC JUNCTION	
Path:	Narrow lumen "obstruction" to high flow
Pt:	Normal patient at normal flow Large diuresis = High flow causes symptoms - Colicky Abdominal Pain - 13 year old on first alcoholic binge that then spontaneously resolves
Dx:	Intravenous Pyelogram (or ultrasound)
Tx:	Stenting Surgery

LOW IMPLANTATION OF THE URETER	
Path:	Ureter—Bladder: Normal Ureter—Urethra: Abnormal
Pt:	Boys—Asymptomatic Girls—"Normal Voiding" AND constant leak
Dx:	Intravenous Pyelogram
Tx:	Reimplantation

VESICOURETERAL REFLUX	
Path:	2-way valves Bacteria ascend
Pt:	Frequent UTIs Or Any pyelo
Dx:	Voiding Cystourethrogram
Tx:	Surgery ... or ... Empiric Antibiotics, Prophylaxis, Wait

CRYPTORCHIDISM	
Path:	Undescended testes
Pt:	Absent testes on physical exam
Dx:	Clinical
Tx:	Newborn: If undescended by 6mo, surgically bring down Prepubertal: Surgically tether Postpubertal: Surgically remove
F/u:	Monitor for testicular cancer ($\uparrow$ 10x risk)

HEMATURIA	
Path:	Unless HUGE trauma, kids don't pee blood
Pt:	Any blood in the urine, microscopic or macroscopic
Dx:	Ultrasound Intravenous Pyelogram ~~CT scan~~ (NEVER! Radiation burden)
Tx:	Congenital Cancer

Urologic Miscellaneous

BPH	
Path:	Enlarged prostate crushes the urethra
Pt:	Urgency, frequency, but NO dysuria Trouble starting, stopping, dribbling, and/or interrupted urine stream Smooth, rubbery prostate (compare to cancer)
Dx:	Urinalysis, Urine Culture (rule out infection) Creatinine Biopsy (NEVER) PSA (NEVER)
Tx:	α-blockers: Tamsulosin, Doxazosin 5-α-reductase-i: Finasteride Foley / In-and-Out post-void residual Surgery (TURP)

ERECTILE DYSFUNCTION	
Path:	Psychiatric or organic
Pt:	Difficulty achieving or maintaining an erection
Dx:	1st: Nighttime Tumescence—to separate psych from organic . . . if it breaks, it's psych, if it doesn't, it's organic
Tx:	Psych: psychotherapy Organic: multiple options, step-wise approach - Injectable Misoprostol (old option) - Phosphodiesterase-I (Sildenafil) - Surgery = Penile Implants

TESTICULAR TORSION	
Path:	Testicle twists, strangulates vascular supply
Pt:	Sudden onset pain without urgency, frequency, or dysuria, without bacteriuria without fever, chills, nausea, vomiting Testicle with Horizontal Lie
Dx:	Clinical . . . Ultrasound with Doppler
Tx:	Surgical: untwist - Pinks up → bilateral orchiopexy - Doesn't → orchiectomy

KIDNEY STONES	
Path:	Obstruction
Pt:	Flank pain + Hematuria
Dx:	CT scan or Ultrasound
Tx:	< 5 mm IVF, Analgesics Between = Lithotripsy > 3 cm Surgical (nephrostomy)
F/u:	24hr-urine, strain for stone

BACTERIAL PROSTATITIS	
Path:	Inflammation of the prostate or infection of the prostate, old men
Pt:	"Pyelo" = Fever, chills, nausea, vomiting, with white blood cells and bacteria Tender prostate on DRE
Dx:	U/A, Urine Culture
Tx:	NEVER REPEAT DRE Bacterial: Fluoroquinolone Not Bacterial: NSAIDs

EPIDIDYMITIS	
Path:	STD (< 40), E.Coli (> 40)
Pt:	Sudden onset pain without urgency, frequency, dysuria. Bacteriuria without fever, chills, nausea, vomiting Testicle in vertical lie Epididymis tender
Dx:	Clinical . . . Ultrasound
Tx:	< 40 Gc/Chla → Ceftriaxone and Doxy > 40 Cipro

Ortho Injury

FRACTURE IN GENERAL	
Path:	Trauma
Dx:	X-rays perpendicular to each other, usually 3 views
Tx:	Open Reduction Internal Fixation - Open - Comminuted - Angular Closed Reduction External Fixation - Closed, closely aligned, or poor surgical candidate

ANTERIOR DISLOCATION OF SHOULDER	
Path:	Minor Trauma (falls, tackle)
Pt:	ADducted EXternally Rotated "Hand Shaking" Position
Dx:	X-ray
Tx:	Set, Sling, Relocate
F/u:	Axillary Nerve = Deltoid Paresthesia

POSTERIOR DISLOCATION OF SHOULDER	
Path:	Major Trauma (seizure, Electrocution)
Pt:	ADducted INternally Rotated Protected Wrist Position
Dx:	X-ray
Tx:	Set, Sling, Relocate
F/u:	Axillary Nerve = Deltoid Paresthesia

COLLES' FRACTURE	
Path:	Osteoporosis Radius "breaks up"
Pt:	Elderly Patient, Osteoporosis Fall onto outstretched hand
Dx:	X-ray = dorsally displaced radius
Tx:	Cast

MONTEGGIA FRACTURE	
Path:	Upward block of a downward blow Ulna Struck first
Pt:	Fractured Ulna Dislocated Radius
Dx:	X-ray
Tx:	ORIF or Casting (severity)

GALEAZZI FRACTURE	
Path:	Downward blow on a pronated arm (radius struck first)
Pt:	Fractured Radius Dislocated Ulna
Dx:	X-ray
Tx:	ORIF or Casting (severity)

BOXER'S FRACTURE	
Path:	Punch misses, hits wall
Pt:	Fracture 4th and 5th Digit
Dx:	X-ray
Tx:	Casting

SCAPHOID FRACTURE	
Path:	Fall onto hand (no Osteoporosis)
Pt:	Young person falls onto hand Hand pain in Snuff Box
Dx:	X-ray = Normal (Day 1) X-ray = Necrosis (Day 3)
Tx:	Cast if Normal X-ray Day 1 ORIF if Fracture on Day 1
F/u:	Tenuous blood supply to distal scaphoid

HIP FRACTURE	
Path:	Major trauma (young) Minor trauma (old, osteoporosis)
Pt:	Leg is shortened and externally rotated
Dx:	X-ray
Tx:	Femoral Head = Hip replacement Intertrochanteric = plates Shaft = Rods ALL ORIF . . . closed for poor surgical candidates
F/u:	Closed fractures = urgent Open fracture = emergent Traction to transport to hospital

Ortho Injury

ACL TEAR	
Path:	Force from BEHIND the knee Leg Locked, Extended when hit
Pt:	Anterior Draw Sign
Dx:	MRI
Tx:	Athletes = Surgical Repair Non-athletes = Conservative

PCL TEAR	
Path:	Force from IN FRONT OF the knee Leg Locked, Extended when hit
Pt:	Posterior Draw Sign
Dx:	MRI
Tx:	Athletes = Surgical Repair Non-athletes = Conservative

COLLATERAL LIGAMENTS	
Path:	Valgus = Lateral Force = Medial Tear Varus = Medial Force = Lateral Tear
Pt:	No buzz phrase, look for injury type (football tackle)
Dx:	MRI
Tx:	One ligament = Hinge Cast Multiple ligament = Surgery

MENISCAL TEAR	
Path:	Uncertain
Pt:	Young, healthy athlete Knee Pain CLICK on full extension
Dx:	MRI . . . only if athlete
Tx:	Athletes = Arthroscopic Repair Non-athletes = Conservative

STRESS FRACTURE	
Path:	Pushing a frail bone beyond capacity
Pt:	Weekend warrior athletes Reserve military forced march Look for "out of shape" and "lots of activity" Pinpoint Tibia pain
Dx:	X-ray = Normal (day 1) X-ray = Fracture (day 7)
Tx:	Cast and crutches even if the x-ray is normal

TIB/FIB FRACTURE	
Path:	Tibia is large, and strong If Tibia breaks, fibular will too

Pt:	Major trauma
	  - Adult pedestrian struck
	  - Purposeful blunt strike to leg
	Deformity often obvious

Dx:	X-ray
Tx:	Closed = Casting Open = ORIF, nailing

ACHILLES TENDON TEAR	
Path:	Avulsion of Achilles Tendon
Pt:	Loud pop → limping Unable to plantar flex foot Gap where the Achilles tendon should be
Dx:	Clinical . . . can use MRI
Tx:	Conservative = Cast (months) Aggressive = Surgery (weeks)

ANKLE FRACTURE, STRAIN, SPRAIN	
Path:	Inversion or Eversion of foot Mechanism: Sprain = Strain = Fracture
Pt:	Swollen, Tender, Painful
Dx:	X-ray to rule out fracture
Tx:	Strain, Sprain = RICE and Crutches Fracture = ORIF or Casting
F/u:	If a person can walk on the foot, do not image

COMPARTMENT SYNDROME	
Path:	Reperfusion Injury Fascial Planes Confined compartment
Pt:	Tense leg Excruciating pain
Dx:	Measure compartment pressures if unsure, surgery if sure
Tx:	Fasciotomy

Ortho Hand

CARPAL TUNNEL	
Path:	Inflammation of the carpal tunnel, compression of the Median nerve
Pt:	↓ Sensation of 1st 3 digits Thenar atrophy Exacerbated by hyperflexion, tapping the carpal tunnel
Dx:	Nerve Conduction Velocity
Tx:	NSAIDs Splinting Steroids Surgery
But:	Treat first, conduction velocity, then surgery

DE QUERVAIN'S TENOSYNOVITIS	
Path:	Tendonitis of the thumb
Pt:	Thumb pain, weight lifter, mom holding baby
Dx:	Fist-Thumb-Twist (Clinical)
Tx:	NSAIDs Splinting + NSAIDS Steroids

JERSEY FINGER	
Path:	Tearing of the flexor tendon
Pt:	When the patient opens his hand, then makes a fist, the finger is unable to flex
Dx:	Clinical
Tx:	Splinting ~~Surgery~~

MALLET FINGER	
Path:	Tearing of the extensor tendon
Pt:	When the patient makes a fist, then opens his hand, the finger is unable to extend
Dx:	Clinical
Tx:	Splinting ~~Surgery~~

TRIGGER FINGER	
Path:	Fascia of the middle finger
Pt:	Unable to flex the middle finger, and a POP with a forced flexion
Dx:	Clinical
Tx:	Steroids

DUPUYTREN'S CONTRACTURE	
Path:	Fascial disease
Pt:	Alcoholic Scandinavian males with a contracted hand and palpable nodules
Dx:	Clinical
Tx:	Surgical Release

FELON	
Path:	Abscess of nail pulp
Pt:	Exquisitely tender Abscess status post penetrating injury Fever and Leukocytosis
Dx:	Clinical
Tx:	Incision and Drainage . . . Antibiotics

Ortho Peds

DEVELOPMENTAL DYSPLASIA OF THE HIP	
Age:	Newborn
Pt:	Clicky hip during the neonatal evaluation, the Ortolani and Barlow maneuvers
Dx:	Ultrasound
Tx:	Harness

LEGG-CALVE-PERTHES	
Age:	6
Pt:	Insidious onset antalgic gait
Dx:	X-ray
Tx:	Cast

SLIPPED-CAPITAL FEMORAL EPIPHYSIS	
Age:	13
Pt:	Fat kid going through a growth spurt. Non-traumatic knee pain
Dx:	Frog-Leg X-ray
Tx:	Surgery

SEPTIC HIP	
Age:	ANY AGE
Pt:	Fever and Joint Pain, especially after another febrile illness or unprotected sex
Dx:	Arthrocentesis
Tx:	Drain and Antibiotics

TRANSIENT SYNOVITIS	
Path:	Post Viral inflammation
Pt:	Hip pain, swelling, weeks after GI or resp virus 0-1 Kocher criteria
Dx:	Clinical
Tx:	Supporive, should resolve in 48 hours

OSGOOD-SCHLATTER'S DISEASE	
Path:	Osteochondrosis
Pt:	Teenage athlete with knee pain, swelling and eventually palpable nodule on the tibia
Dx:	Clinical
Tx:	Rest + Cast (aka stop exercising, curative) Work through it (palpable nodule)

SCOLIOSIS	
Path:	Deformity of the spine
Pt:	Teenage girl who can present with either moderate: cosmetic severe: shortness of breath
Dx:	Adam's Test is positive (have the girl lean forward and see asymmetry)
Tx:	No therapy Brace Surgery with rods

BONE TUMOR—EWING'S SARCOMA	
Path:	Ewing = t11,22 midshaft
Pt:	Bone pain
Dx:	1st: X-ray shows midshaft lesion with onion-skin pattern Then: MRI Best: Biopsy, resection
Tx:	Surgery

BONE TUMOR—OSTEOSARCOMA	
Path:	Retinoblastoma gene, associated with retinoblastoma of the eye
Pt:	Kid who had retinoblastoma of the eye who presents with bone pain
Dx:	1st: X-ray shows end-of-the-bone lesion with sunburst pattern Then: MRI Best: Biopsy, resection
Tx:	Surgery

FRACTURE IN KIDS	
Path:	Fractures can occur for any reason, trauma, fall, and child abuse. You must think of the growth plate, a consideration not in adults
Pt:	Leg pain, trauma
Dx:	X-ray
Tx:	Involves growth plate → ORIF Does not involve growth plate → Cast

Shock—Step 2 Requires Very Little Here

HEMORRHAGE = HYPOVOLEMIC	
Path:	Decreased Preload, Volume down from bleeding
Pt:	Flat neck veins ↓ Hemoglobin / ↓ Hematocrit
Dx:	FAST = U/S
Tx:	Plug the hole and give blood 2 large bore IVs, type and cross, transfuse

TENSION PNEUMOTHORAX = OBSTRUCTIVE	
Path:	Decreased preload Air compresses vena cava, backs up blood before the RIGHT ventricle
Pt:	Engorged neck veins Tracheal Deviation Hyperresonant lungs
Dx:	~~CXR~~ (DON'T WAIT, ACT!)
Tx:	Needle decompression Thoracostomy (chest tube)

PERICARDIAL TAMPONADE = OBSTRUCTIVE	
Path:	Rapidly evolving or large pericardial effusion Decreased preload Backs blood up before the RIGHT ventricle
Pt:	Engorged Neck Veins Distant heart Sounds Normal Lungs Pulsus Paradoxus > 10 mm Hg
Dx:	FAST = Ultrasound
Tx:	Pericardiocentesis

CONTRACTILITY = CARDIOGENIC	
Path:	Decreased ejection fraction Backs up blood before the LEFT ventricle
Pt:	Engorged neck veins Pulmonary Edema
Dx:	FAST = Echo = Ultrasound
Tx:	Medical Management

VASOMOTOR SHOCK = DISTRIBUTIVE	
Path:	Loss of vasomotor tone Dysfunctional ANS . . . anaphylaxis, sepsis, spinal trauma, anesthesia, etc.
Pt:	Warm extremities, low BP
Dx:	Underlying disease specific
Tx:	Vasopressors (fluid first)

TRADITIONAL SHOCK COMPARED TO OURS	
Preload	Hypovolemic
Contractility and HR	Cardiogenic
Preload	Obstructive
-------------------------	----------------------
SVR	Distributive

OUR WAY OF DOING IT		

$$CO \qquad X \qquad SVR$$
$$/ \quad \backslash$$
$$HR \quad SV$$
$$/ \quad \backslash$$
$$Preload \quad Contractility$$

Heart Rate:	Too Fast Too Slow
Preload:	Volume ↓: - Diarrhea - Dehydration - Diuresis - Hemorrhage ↓ Preload - Tension Pneumo - Tamponade - The PE
Contractility	MI CHF
SVR	Sepsis Anaphylaxis Neurogenic Spinal Anesthesia Addison's Disease

Head Trauma

BASILAR SKULL FRACTURE	
Path:	Fracture of the base of the skull
Pt:	Raccoon eyes (ecchymosis around the eyes) Battle Signs (ecchymosis behind ears) Clear rhinorrhea / otorrhea (CSF)
Dx:	CT scan
Tx:	Surgical repair

EPIDURAL HEMATOMA	
Path:	Rupture of the middle meningeal artery
Pt:	Walk-Talk-And-Die. Major trauma to the side of head with loss of consciousness, lucid period, then they die.
Dx:	CT scan showing a lens shaped hematoma
Tx:	Craniectomy

ACUTE SUBDURAL HEMATOMA	
Path:	Rupture of the bridging veins
Pt:	Shaken baby syndrome (pediatric), who suffer trauma, goes into a coma, and dies
Dx:	CT scan = crescent shaped hematoma
Tx:	↓ ICP = Elevate the head of the bed, hyperventilate, mannitol, ventriculostomy

CHRONIC SUBDURAL HEMATOMA	
Path:	Tearing of the bridging veins
Pt:	Older, fall trauma. Look for alcoholic / progressive dementia.
Dx:	CT scan = crescent
Tx:	Craniotomy

CONCUSSION	
Path:	Bruising of the brain
Pt:	Head trauma Possible LoC Possible amnesia Grading concussions
Dx:	CT scan = normal
Tx:	Stabilize C-spine and airway if needed Do not let athlete return to play Cognitive + physical rest needed with gradual return

DIFFUSE AXONAL INJURY	
Path:	Edema of cortex / cord
Pt:	Angular trauma (almost always vehicular) that progresses into coma.
Dx:	CT scan = Blurring of grey-white junction
Tx:	Supportive, severity of injury correlates with duration of coma

Neck Trauma

Upper Zone   Arteriogram

Middle Zone   Safely Explored

Basal Zone   Esophagram,
              Bronchogram,
              Arteriogram

STAB WOUNDS		
Hematoma, gurgling, shock		Surgery
Upper Zone	Asx	Observe → CT or U/S
Middle Zone	Asx	Observe → CT or U/S
Basal Zone	Asx	CXR or CT → Observe

GUN SHOTS		
Hematoma, gurgling, shock		Surgery
Upper Zone	Asx	CT or U/S → Surgery
Middle Zone	Asx	CT or U/S → Surgery
Basal Zone	Asx	CT → Surgery

COMPLETE TRANSECTION OF THE CORD
Motor, pain, and vibration are lost below the site of the lesion
Lower motor neuron sxs at the level of lesion and upper motor neuron sxs below.
All lesions are bilateral.

HEMISECTION	
Path:	Stabbing
Pt:	Ipsilateral loss of motor— upper motor neuron sxs below, lower motor neuron sxs at lesion Contralateral loss of pain Ipsilateral loss of vibratory sense

CENTRAL CORD SYNDROME
Old person in a severe motor vehicle accident
Hyperextension of the neck, narrowing of the cord already
Loss of pain and temperature
May be motor loss as well (usually recovers)

Chest Trauma

RIB FRACTURE	
Path:	Blunt trauma to chest
Pt:	Pain, tender and pleuritic Patient may not inhale deeply
Dx:	CXR
Tx:	Opiates ~~Binders~~
F/u:	Caution Atelectasis → Pneumonia Rib Fractures cause penetrating trauma

PNEUMOTHORAX	
Path:	Penetrating trauma Air fills pleural space
Pt:	Shortness of breath, hyperresonance, and decreased lung sounds
Dx:	CXR shows vertical lung shadow
Tx:	Chest Tube (thoracostomy)
F/u:	If JVD and Hypotension, it is a tension pneumothorax . . . do needle decompression

HEMOTHORAX	
Path:	Penetrating trauma Blood fills the pleural space
Pt:	Shortness of breath, decreased lung sounds, dullness to percussion
Dx:	CXR shows horizontal lung shadow; air fluid level
Tx:	Chest Tube (thoracostomy)
F/u:	1500 cc on insertion or 600 cc/6hours prompts surgical exploration = thoracotomy

SUCKING CHEST WOUND	
Path:	Penetrating trauma
Pt:	Flap of skin allows for air to enter on inhalation, but not out on exhalation
Pt:	Same as pneumothorax, likely to produce a tension pneumo
Tx:	Occlusive dressing taped on 3 sides
F/u:	Needle decompression if tension pneumo

FLAIL CHEST	
Path:	Blunt trauma Two or more ribs broken in two or more places such that ribs move paradoxically with respiration (out on exhale)
Pt:	Paradoxical wall motion on respiration
Dx:	Chest X-ray
Tx:	Keep the ribs in alignment so they heal
F/u:	Marker for severe trauma— pulmonary / cardiac contusion, aortic dissection

PULMONARY CONTUSION	
Path:	Severe, massive blunt trauma Contused lungs leak = pulmonary edema Suspect if scapular fracture, sternal fracture or flail chest
Pt:	24-48 hours after trauma shortness of breath and pulmonary edema
Dx:	Chest X-ray, white out when it was normal day one
Tx:	Treat as heart failure: - Avoid large volume fluids - Diuresis, gentle

MYOCARDIAL CONTUSION	
Path:	Severe, massive blunt trauma Contused heart = non-vascular MI Suspect if scapular fracture, sternal fracture or flail chest
Pt:	Severe trauma. Do NOT rely on chest pain, anticipate and actively look for this
Dx:	ECGs and Troponins
Tx:	MONA BASH

TRAUMATIC DISSECTION OF AORTA	
Path:	Severe, massive blunt trauma Ligamentum Arteriosum tears aorta Suspect if scapular fracture, sternal fracture flail chest, or deformed steering wheel
Pt:	Dead on scene Asymptomatic until the patient dies
Dx:	Prophylactic Chest x-ray shows mediastinum widening CT Angiogram of the Chest
Tx:	Anti-hypertensives Surgical Repair

TRAUMA SURG

Abdominal Trauma

PENETRATING TRAUMA	
GSW:	Below T4 (nipple) = Ex Lap Run the bowel DO NOT remove the bullet Exception (small caliber bullets that do not get into peritoneum)

Stab:	Evisceration = Ex Lap
	Hemodynamic Instability = Ex Lap
	Peritoneal Signs = Ex Lap
	
	Exception (wound that does not
	    penetrate peritoneum. Start by
	    exploring the wound, then FAST
	    exam)

BLUNT TRAUMA	
Path:	Find hemorrhage
Dx:	FAST CT scan if stable ~~Diagnostic Peritoneal Lavage~~
Tx:	Ex Lap See the next sections

SPLENIC LACERATION	
Path:	Non-vital, serves immune Bleeds (a lot) Has a capsule
Tx:	Repair if able Splenectomy if necessary
F/u:	Vaccinations against encapsulated organism

LIVER LACERATION	
Path:	Vital organ Bleeds A lot Has a capsule Most common cause of intra- abdominal hemorrhage
Tx:	Lobectomy as needed Pringle Maneuver to control bleeding (hepatoduodenal ligament)

RUPTURED DIAPHRAGM	
Path:	Non-vital, No Capsule, Non-bleeder
Pt:	Bowel sounds in the chest Kehr's Sign = shoulder pain
Dx:	Chest X-ray
Tx:	Surgical Repair

PELVIC FRACTURES	

Path:	High-speed, large-damage (MVA,
	    falls)
	Pelvic Fractures are the gateway
	    injury

Pt:	+ Hip-rocking + Crepitus, + Pelvic Floor Instability
Dx:	CT scan
Tx:	Externally fix the hip, allow to heal
F/u:	Pelvic hematoma (below)

PELVIC INJURIES: URETHRAL INJURY	
Path:	Pelvic fracture
Pt:	Blood at meatus High-Riding Prostate
Dx:	Intravenous Pyelogram
Tx:	Surgery Suprapubic Catheter . . . NO FOLEY

PELVIC INJURIES: RECTAL INJURY	
Path:	Pelvic fracture
Pt:	Bloody Diarrhea Bowel Dysfunction
Dx:	Proctoscope
Tx:	Surgery

PELVIC HEMATOMA	
Path:	Pelvic fracture
Pt:	Decreasing Hemoglobin
Dx:	Hemoglobin drops CT Scan
Tx:	Transfuse. Do NOT explore IR-guided embolization

Burns

SEVERITY OF BURNS	
1st :	Epidermis, Erythema
2nd:	Dermis, Erythema, + Blisters
3rd:	Dermis or deeper, painless white/ charred center, surrounded by 2nd degree burns

CHEMICAL BURNS	
Path:	Alkaline burns are worse than acidic burns
Pt:	Any contact with a chemical
Tx:	Irrigation is crucial . . . flush . . . flush . . . flush
F/u:	If ingested, DO NOT induce vomiting Ingest a mild buffer

ELECTRICAL BURNS	
Path:	Lightning strikes High-voltage lines
Pt:	Entrance and exit wounds Cardiac arrest
F/u:	Check a CK level for Rhabdo If Rhabdo, give fluids—lots of fluids Posterior Shoulder Dislocations Demyelination Syndromes

RESPIRATORY BURNS	
Path:	Burns to the mouth Inhalation injury of smoke or hot gas
Pt:	Trapped indoors during a fire Soot in mouth / nose Singed facial hair
Dx:	Bronchoscopy if high risk
Tx:	Intubation

CIRCUMFERENTIAL BURNS	
Path:	Burns around an extremity Edema causes compression of vessels
Pt:	Thick, leathery Eschar
Dx:	Clinical
Tx:	Cut the Eschar
F/u:	Concern for Compartment Syndrome

BURN CARE	
Fluid:	(Kg BW x % BSA Burned x 4 cc) = replacement . . . Parkland Formula
Goal:	Urine Output Blood Pressure
Wound:	Silver Sulfadiazine
Rehab:	Early mobilization (painful)

TRAUMA SURG

Bites

RABIES	
Path:	Animal Bite If domesticated → observe If wild animal → kill and biopsy If wild animal but cannot catch → IgG and Vaccine If biopsy positive → IgG and Vaccine If biopsy negative → reassure patient

SNAKEBITES	
Path:	Slit-like eyes, rattlers, cobra cowl
Pt:	Erythema, Skin changes, pain at bite site
Tx:	Anti-venom NO cutting NO sucking NO tourniqueting

BEE STINGS	
1	If non-allergic, remove pincer, monitor There are no venomous properties
2	If anaphylaxis, 1:1000 SubQ epi Follow with antihistamines and steroids if needed

3	Urticaria at the site of the sting
	    without any other sign of
	    anaphylaxis warrants monitoring

BLACK WIDOW SPIDER BITES	
Path:	Black Spider, Hourglass on its belly
Pt:	Abdominal Pain, N/V, Pancreatitis
Tx:	IV Calcium

BROWN RECLUSE	
Path:	Attic, Old Boxes, South
Pt:	Necrotic ulcer with ring of erythema
Tx:	Wide Debridement, skin grafts

HUMAN BITES	
Path:	Sexual Encounters, Fist fight
Pt:	Laceration only, cover story
Tx:	If local and not severe: irrigate and oral abx
Wound:	If extensive or severe: surgical exploration

Toxic Ingestion

CARBON MONOXIDE	
Path:	Carbon Monoxide binds hemoglobin better than oxygen
Pt:	Cherry-red skin, confusion, headaches Singes nose hairs Smoke inhalation injuries
Dx:	ABG = Carboxyhemoglobin SpO_2 100%, but ABG shows ↓ PaO_2
Tx:	100% Oxygen Track Carboxyhemoglobin

ACETAMINOPHEN	
Path:	Hepatotoxic
Pt:	Fulminant hepatic failure Either suicidal (intentional) or chronic pain (unintentional)
Dx:	Acetaminophen Nomogram
Tx:	N-Acetyl-Cysteine

ETHYLENE GLYCOL	
Path:	Anti-freeze Metabolites turn toxic
Pt:	Alcoholic, renal failure ↑ Anion Gap AND ↑ Osmolar Gap
Dx:	Urinalysis = Envelope-Shaped Calcium Crystals Wood's Lamp of urine = lights up (Fluorescein dye in Antifreeze)
Tx:	Fomepizole >> EtOH Dialysis

METHEMOGLOBIN	
Path:	HIV drugs
Pt:	SpO_2 88% but ABG shows normal PaO_2
Dx:	Methemoglobin level
Tx:	Methylene Blue

ORGANOPHOSPHATES	
Path:	Acetylcholinesterase Inhibition
Pt:	Farmer with pesticides, Chemical Plant, Soldier Exposed in Battle SLUDGE = Salivation, Lacrimation, Urination, Defecation, GI upset, Emesis
Dx:	Clinical
Tx:	Treat yourself and others = decontamination Treat the patient = Atropine Treat the poison = 2-PAM

See Psychiatry for Intoxication and Withdrawal from drugs of addiction. See Burns for chemical ingestion.

Prevention

LEVELS OF PREVENTION	
Primary	Prevent **onset** of dz Vaccines, diet/exercise
Secondary	Prevent **progression** of dz Screening, hypertension meds
Tertiary	Prevent **complications** of dz Surgery, rehab
All medicine falls under 1 of these 3.	

Screening

CANCER		
Colon	50-75	Colonoscopy q10y Flex Sig q5y+FOBT q3y FOTB q1y
Breast	40-49	if + family history only (BRCA1/2)
	50-74	Mammo q2y
Cervical	21-65	Pap Smear q3y
Lung	55-80 + 30 pack-yr + Quit < 15 yrs	Low Dose CT q1y

MEDICAL DISEASES		
Cholesterol	♀ 45, ♂ 35, 20 if at risk	Fasting Lipid Panel q5y
Htn	Everybody	Check BP every visit
DM	Htn	A1c ~~2 hr GTT~~
HLD	♂ > 35, > 25 if RF ♀ > 45, > 25 if RF	Lipid Panel (statins)
Osteoporosis	♀ 65 (high risk at 60)	One time dexa scan
AAA	♂ 65-75 yrs + smoke	One-time U/S of abdominal aorta
STDs	Sexually Active	Rapid tests at least once, pref q1y
Hepatitis C	Baby Boomers	One time antibody screen
Depression	All adults	PHQ9, clinical judgement
Alcohol misuse	All adults	Interview

Vaccinations

VACCINE—WHEN—WHO		
Tdap	q10y x 3 doses See "treating a wound" below	Everybody
Pneumo	13 as kid, 23 ≥ 65	For 23, all ≥ 65, at risk (comorbid dz) < 65
Zoster	Once > 60	Everybody
Hep A/B	3 doses in 6 months (start at birth)	Everybody
Meningo	2 doses (11+16)	College, travel
HPV	♂ and ♀ before sexually active (9-13) 3 doses over 6 months	Everybody
MMRV	2 doses (@1&4)	All children
HiB	4 doses in 1st year	All < 5
Flu	Annually	Everybody

VACCINE CONTRAINDICATIONS	
All	Anaphylaxis (i.e., allergic to gelatin)
Flu (live)	Egg Allergy (give recombinant inactive instead)
Live	↓ Immune

MANAGING A WOUND WITH < 3 LIFETIME DOSES (OR UNKNOWN)	
Type of Wound	
Clean	Dirty
Tdap	Tdap +TIG
TIMING DOESN'T MATTER IF < 3 Lifetime Doses	

MANAGING A WOUND WITH ≥ 3 LIFETIME DOSES	
Type of Wound	
Clean	Dirty
≥ 10y Tdap	≥ 5y Tdap
< 10y Home	< 5y Home
No TIG needed if ≥ 3 lifetime doses	

Diagnostic Tests

2X2 TABLE		
	Disease	
Test or Exposure	+	-
+	A	B
-	C	D
A:	True Positive	
B:	False Positive	
C:	False Negative	
D:	True Negative	

DIAGNOSTIC TESTS	
Sensitivity	A / A + C Ability to detect true positives
Specificity	D / B + D Ability to confirm true negatives
PPV	A / A + B Probability of disease in pt with + test result, ↑ prevalence ↑ PPV
NPV	D / C + D Probability of no disease in pt with − test result, ↑ prevalence ↓ NPV

Study Design

EXPERIMENTAL STUDY	
Randomized Controlled Trial	Gold standard, uses intervention vs. control groups & tracks dz outcomes, uses odds ratio
Intervention	= The treatment
Control	= Placebo / Standard of Care / Nothing

OBSERVATIONAL STUDIES	
Case Series	Qualitative, narrative
Cross Sectional	Retrospective, snapshot of dz and exposure in a given time, uses prevalence
Cohort	Prospective, starts with exposed vs. unexposed and tracks dz outcomes over time, uses relative risk
Case Control	Retrospective, starts with dz vs. no dz and looks at exposures, uses odds ratio
Observational studies can't establish causation (only correlation)	

METHODS TO ELIMINATE BIAS	
Randomization	Blinding
Standardization	Statistical Controlling
Bias is addressed in study design.	

Bias

BIAS IN STUDIES/SCREENS	
Lead Time	Pt awareness of diagnosis changes, but no effect on outcome, artificially ↑ survival time
Length Time	Deadly dz is found less often, bias that assumes finding dz means it's less dangerous, artificially makes screening ↑
Overdiagnosis	Diagnosis is ↑ but has Ø effect on mortality, is meaningless. Artificially ↑ survival stats
Selection	Pt group isn't chosen at random, can't get meaningful comparisons, skews outcome
Measurement	Using different tools to measure same thing, can't get meaningful comparisons, skews outcome
Recall	Sick patients remember more, skews risk outcomes
Information	Pts know something that affects their actions, skews outcome
Observer	Knowing being observed leads to change in pt behaviors, skews reliability
Publication	Null/negative results less likely to be published, skews available data
Confounding	3rd variable that has a noncasual relationship with exposure AND outcome, why correlation doesn't = causation

Hypothesis Testing

GROUP 1 VS. GROUP 2	
H_o	Group 1 = Group 2 (what we test)
H_a	Group 1 ≠ Group 2 (what we want)
α	α = significance level (.05). 5% chance difference is due to random chance alone
P value	**If P < α, can reject H_o**

TYPES OF ERROR		
	H_o True	H_o False
Guess H_o T	Correct	Type 2 error (β, false -)
Guess H_o F	Type 1 error (α, false +)	Correct

Confidence Interval

ASSOCIATIONS	
Null	CI includes 1
Effect Size	Furthest from 1
Power	Narrowest range

Risk

2X2 TABLE			
	Disease		
Exposure		+	-
	+	A	B
	-	C	D
A:	True Positive		
B:	False Positive		
C:	False Negative		
D:	True Negative		

RISK MEASUREMENTS	
Odds Ratio (Case-Control)	(A x D) / (B x C) Measure of association, case control study (i.e., pt with Dz 5x more likely to have Ex)
Relative Risk (Cohort)	(A / (A + B)) / (C / (C + D)) Measure of association, cohort study (i.e., pt with Ex 5x more likely to have Dz)